THE LAST GIFT:

The Conversation That Prevents Family Trauma

By

Donnett Sinclair, RN, MSN, MBA

The Last Gift

By Donnett Sinclair, RN, MSN, MBA

The Last Gift Annual Review™ is a trademark of Donnett Sinclair.

 ISBN: 979-8-9946100-0-8

Published by: Donnett Sinclair, Atlanta, GA.

Book design by: Abdul Rehman

Cover design by: Majid Khan

First Edition

DISCLAIMER

While the author has made every effort to provide accurate phone numbers, internet addresses, and other contact details at the time of publication, neither the publisher nor the author assumes responsibility for any errors or changes that occur after publication. Additionally, the publisher does not control or assume responsibility for any author or third-party websites or their content.

This book is not intended to replace professional medical, legal, or psychological advice. The information provided is for educational and informational purposes only. Readers should consult qualified healthcare professionals, attorneys, and counselors about their specific situations and needs. The author and publisher explicitly disclaim any liability, loss, or risk resulting directly or indirectly from the use or application of any content in this book.

The stories and examples in this book come from the author's twenty years of hospice nursing experience. Names, identifying details, and certain circumstances have been changed to protect patients' and families' privacy. Some stories are composites of multiple cases. Any resemblance to specific individuals, living or dead, is purely coincidental.

Printed in the United States of America

DEDICATION

For my husband, Horace, who showed me that hope and preparation are not opposites; they are both acts of love.

You fought End Stage Renal Disease for eight years with resilience and grace. You never gave up hope, and you never shied away from the truth. That courage, to face death while still fighting for life, saved me from a trauma worse than grief alone. This book is your legacy.

And for every family that has ever sat in a hospital room at 2 AM, tormented by the question: "What would they have wanted?" For every spouse who has faced impossible decisions alone, wondering forever if they did the right thing. For every parent who left this world without sharing their wishes, leaving behind confusion and regret. For every person who thought, "We have more time," until suddenly, they didn't.

This book is for you.

May we learn to discuss death as openly as we discuss birth. May we plan for our passing with the same care we take for our lives. May we give our families the gift my husband gave me: certainty, clarity, and peace. May we complete the circle.

In loving memory of a man who never stopped fighting but also never avoided the truth.

I miss you every day.

Table of Contents

PROLOGUE

Why I Had to Write This Book

He stopped breathing by the time we reached the emergency department.

That Sunday morning, I sensed something was wrong. He was overly sleepy. Too quiet. When I suggested it was time for his home dialysis, he shook his head, too exhausted to respond. I checked his blood pressure. It was lower than usual. Much lower.

"We need to go to the hospital," I told him. He didn't argue. That's when I realized he felt worse than he was letting on.

His best friend drove. I sat in the back seat with my husband, holding him close, rubbing his forehead the way he liked. His eyes were closed. His breathing was shallow.

"We're almost there," I kept saying. "Just a few more minutes."

I'm a hospice nurse. I've watched hundreds of people die. I recognize labored breathing. I understand what "too sleepy" means for someone with end-stage renal disease. But when it's your husband, you tell yourself a different story.

This is just another admission. They'll stabilize him. We'll get through this.

We arrived at the emergency entrance. His friend parked. I opened the door.

"Honey, we're here. Can you walk?"

No response.

"Honey?"

His chest wasn't moving.

"He's not breathing! Help! We need help now!"

1

They rushed him inside. And with the certainty that comes from twenty years of watching people die, I knew this time was different.

This wasn't just another admission. This was the end.

My husband lived with end-stage renal disease for eight years. Eight years of dialysis. Eight years of hospitalizations so predictable I could anticipate the sequence. Eight years of hoping for a transplant that never came. Eight years of telling ourselves we had more time.

I knew ESRD was terminal. I knew the trajectory. I had cared for countless patients. dying from it. I understood what "end stage" meant. But when it was my husband, I believed something different. "He's resilient." "We're going to beat this." "A transplant will come."

He would state it firmly: "I'm not going anywhere."

And I believed him, not because the evidence supported it, but because believing was safer than facing the truth. Because hope felt better than preparation. Because denial, even for a hospice nurse, is powerful. And yet, despite all of that, we had the conversation.

Three years earlier, on a quiet Sunday afternoon, I asked him what he would want if something happened. He told me clearly, without hesitation. He wanted to be cremated, with his ashes scattered in the Caribbean Sea in Jamaica, where he was from. He said he wanted Bob Marley's music playing at his celebration of life; any Bob Marley song would do. "I love anything from Bob." He didn't want an open casket. I asked, "Your mother believes in seeing the body. Have you talked to her about that?" He paused, "I did once, but I need to have that conversation with her again." He asked me to deliver his eulogy, and I agreed. We talked about quality of life. He made it clear: if he was in a vegetative state with no chance of recovery, he wanted only comfort care; no machines to keep him alive artificially. "I want to go with dignity," he said. "Not hooked up to tubes for months." I nodded, treasuring every word like precious cargo. The conversation lasted about thirty minutes, then we went back to our usual Sunday—grocery shopping, watching a movie, living our lives.

When he died, two hours after we arrived at the hospital, I was devastated. But I didn't need to guess. I understood what he wanted when the doctor asked about life support. I knew how to organize his memorial. I knew how to honor him, even as it tore me apart.

That conversation became the greatest gift he ever gave me.

For over twenty years, I told families, "Have the conversation while you still can." And still, I convinced myself I had more time. That is the brutal truth: If a hospice nurse can live in denial, anyone can.

We avoid these conversations not because we lack love for our families, but because we believe silence protects them. However, it doesn't. Silence leaves them guessing, burdens them with guilt, and turns grief into trauma.

This book exists because a single thirty-minute conversation, held years before death, can save the people you love from unbearable uncertainty. Hope and planning are not mutually exclusive. You can believe in miracles and still take prepared actions. You can fight for life and still make plans for death. This book will show you how.

PART ONE:

WHY THIS MATTERS

CHAPTER 1:

How Death Moved from Bedroom to Hospital (And What We Lost)

When I entered Room 437 at 2 AM, I immediately understood what I was witnessing: a peaceful death turning into a nightmare. Mr. Johnson was actively dying. I'd been a hospice nurse long enough to recognize the signs: mottled hands, irregular breathing with long pauses, the barely-there pulse. He'd be gone within hours, maybe minutes.

But the room was chaotic.

His wife stood at the bedside, yelling at the attending physician: "Do something! Give him more oxygen! Don't just stand there! Don't let him die!" His 45-year-old son, red-faced and trembling, jabbed his finger at the nurse: "The second his heart stops, you perform CPR. Do you hear me? You do NOT give up on him!" His daughter sat in the corner, sobbing uncontrollably: "I don't know what he wanted. We never talked about this. I don't know what to do!"

The attending physician looked at me with exhausted, desperate eyes. I'd seen that look before. No advance directive. No documented wishes. No healthcare proxy. Nothing.

Mr. Johnson had been admitted three days earlier with end-stage heart failure. His kidneys were shutting down, his lungs filling with fluid, his body shutting down in the way bodies do when they've reached their limit. His cardiologist had tried to have "the talk" that afternoon: "Mr. Johnson's body is failing. We need to discuss what he'd want if his heart stops." But the family shut it down immediately. "He's a fighter! Don't talk about giving up!" "He's going to pull through this!" "We're not discussing death!" So now here we were at 2 AM with Mr. Johnson unconscious and unable to speak for himself, while his family tore each other apart.

I pulled the physician aside in the hallway. "Does he have a DNR?" "No. Family refused to discuss it." "Living will?" "Nothing on file." "Healthcare power of attorney?" "The wife says she's his proxy, but there's no legal document. And the son is threatening to sue us if we 'let his father die.'"

I closed my eyes. I'd seen this scene play out a hundred times.

Back in the room, the fighting continued. The son to his mother: "If you tell them not to do CPR, you're killing him!" The mother to her son: "Don't you dare talk to me that way! I know what's best for your father!" The daughter: "Please stop fighting! Please! I just want to know what Dad would want!"

But none of them knew because they'd never asked.

At 3:17 AM, Mr. Johnson's heart stopped.

The son screamed, "Do CPR! NOW!"

For the next 45 minutes, we performed chest compressions on an 82-year-old man whose body had been shutting down for days. We broke his ribs—I heard them crack under my hands. We shocked his heart repeatedly. We pumped him full of medications. His wife stood in the corner, watching in horror. His daughter vomited in the hallway. His son demanded we keep going.

At 4:02 AM, the attending physician declared him dead. Mr. Johnson was gone, and his family was shattered.

Later, in the hallway, as his wife sobbed and his children stood in stunned silence, I heard the son tell his sister: "We killed him. We didn't do enough. We gave up on him."

And I heard his sister tell their mother, "We tortured him, all that CPR. We should have let him go peacefully. I'll never forgive myself."

And I overheard the mother say to no one in particular, "I don't know what he wanted. Fifty-seven years of marriage, and I don't know what he wanted."

One family. Destroyed. Not just by death, but by the preventable trauma of silence.

Two weeks later, I ran into the daughter at the grocery store. She looked like she hadn't slept since her father died.

"We're not speaking," she told me quietly. "My brother and I. He thinks we killed Dad by not doing more. I think we tortured Dad by doing too much. My mother is caught in the middle, guilt-ridden and paralyzed."

She paused, tears streaming down her face.

"If he'd just told us what he wanted. If we'd just asked. If we'd had one conversation..."

I held her hand. "I'm so sorry," I said because I was. And because I knew: this was preventable.

How We Got Here

Mr. Johnson's death, chaotic, traumatic, and tearing his family apart, isn't unusual. It's the norm in 21st-century America. But it wasn't always this way. To understand how death became something we don't talk about, don't plan for, and handle so catastrophically, we need to go back to a time when death looked completely different. Back to 1900, when most Americans died at home, surrounded by family, with everyone knowing what was happening and what to expect. Back to when death was a family event, not a medical crisis. Back to before death moved from the bedroom to the hospital, and what we lost in that transition.

Death In 1900: The Home Death

In 1900, if you asked an American where people died, they'd look at you strangely. "At home, of course. Where else would they die?" In 1900, 85% of Americans died at home. Not because home was necessarily better, but because there was no alternative. Hospitals were for surgery and acute illness. Dying happened at home. What did that look like? When someone was dying:

Grandmother's breathing changes. She's been bedridden for three days, her consumption (tuberculosis) reaching its final stage. The family gathers. Children are sent to fetch relatives from neighboring farms. Within hours, everyone arrives: siblings, cousins, neighbors. They take turns sitting with Grandmother, wiping her brow, holding her hand, reading Bible verses, and singing hymns.

The children watch. They've seen this before. Death isn't hidden from them; it's part of life. They've seen baby chicks die, farm animals slaughtered, and now they witness their grandmother's final hours.

The local midwife or doctor stops by, although there's little they can do. "Keep her comfortable," they say. "She won't be long now."

Grandmother dies at 4 PM on a Tuesday, in her own bed, surrounded by three generations of family.

What happens next:

Her daughters wash her body, dress her in her Sunday best, and place coins on her eyelids to keep them closed. They move her to the parlor, laying her in a simple wooden coffin built by a local carpenter. For two days, the community pays respects. Neighbors bring food. People tell stories. Children peek at the body, their first close encounter with death.

On Thursday, after a simple service in the parlor, six men carried the coffin to the family cemetery plot. She's buried near her husband, her parents, and her infant son, who died thirty years earlier. Everyone was involved. Everyone knew what was happening. Death was a family event.

What 1900 Families Knew

By 1900, the average person had experienced multiple deaths by the age of 10.

- Siblings (infant mortality was high)
- Grandparents (usually died at home)
- Neighbors, church members, community members
- Farm animals (death was visible on farms)

Death literacy was high because death was visible.

Children learned:

- What dying looks like (the physical changes)
- What to do when someone dies (family rituals)
- How to grieve (community mourning practices)
- That death was natural, inevitable, and part of life

Nobody needed a handbook on "how to support a dying person." They had seen it dozens of times.

The Shift: 1945-1970

Then everything shifted. Between 1945 and 1970, death moved from the home to the hospital.

What caused the shift:

1. Medical advances

- Antibiotics (1940s) – suddenly, infections became curable.
- Better surgeries, hospitals became places of healing rather than places of death.
- Intensive care units (1950s-60s) could keep people alive longer.
- Ventilators, feeding tubes, and life support.

2. Urbanization

- Families migrated to urban areas.
- Smaller homes (no space for dying or dead in apartments)
- Nuclear families (not multi-generational households)
- Less community support

3. Professionalization of death

- Hospitals took charge of the dying.
- Funeral homes have taken over death care, which was previously handled by families.
- Doctors became "death experts" (replacing family knowledge)

4. Cultural shift

- Death is regarded as a medical failure
- Fight death instead of accepting it.
- Death turned into "hospital business," not a "family event."

By 1980, 75% of Americans died in hospitals or institutions, marking a complete reversal over 80 years.

WHAT WE LOST

When death moved from home to hospital, we lost more than just the setting. We lost death literacy.

In 1900, a 10-year-old knew:

- What dying looks like
- How to sit with someone who's dying
- What to do when someone dies
- How to grieve in community

In 2000, a 40-year-old might have never:

- Seen someone die
- Touched a dead body

- Witnessed the dying process
- Learned family death rituals

Death became invisible. Hidden. Something "professionals" handle.

We lost family involvement.

In 1900, Families washed the body, prepared the burial, held vigil, and buried their loved ones themselves.

In 2000, Funeral homes picked up the body. Professionals take care of everything. Families come for a brief viewing and ceremony.

Death became something done TO families, not BY families. We lost the ability to plan for death.

In 1900, Everyone knew how people in their community died, what to expect, and what the family would do.

In 2000, no one discussed death until the crisis happened. Then families hurried, guessed, and argued. Planning shifted from prudent to "morbid."

We lost our community traditions.

In 1900, the entire community gathered. Rituals were clear, and everyone knew their role.

In 2000, isolated nuclear families managed on their own, without shared rituals. Each family figured everything out independently.

Grief became privatized, Lonely.

The Result: The Johnson Family

This leads us back to Mr. Johnson's death at 2 AM in Room 437. Why was it so traumatic? Not because he died; death is inevitable.

But because:

- His family had never encountered death firsthand.
- They didn't understand what death looks like.
- They never discussed his wishes.
- They had no plan, preparation, or framework.
- They were taught: "Don't talk about death."
- When the crisis hit, they were completely unprepared.

And so, a natural death turned into a trauma. CPR that broke ribs. Family members shouting at each other. Guilt that will haunt them for years. Relationships withered away. All avoidable. All the result of death moving from the bedroom to the hospital, and taking death literacy with it.

Where We Are Now (2025)

The statistics:

- 60% of Americans die in hospitals or nursing homes.
- 70% say they want to die at home (but only 30% do).
- 90% believe that advance care planning is important, but only 30% have advance directives.

Most families have never discussed end-of-life wishes.

Average hospice stays are 18 days, which is too short; the ideal duration is 2-3 months.

We have created a culture that denies death, where:

- Talking about death is labeled as "morbid."
- Planning for death is viewed as "giving up."
- Dying in a hospital hooked to machines is considered "normal."
- Family trauma is seen as "unavoidable."

However, it's not unavoidable. It is the predictable outcome of a lack of death literacy.

The Good News

We can reclaim what we've lost not by going back to 1900 (since no one wants death without modern medicine), but by reclaiming:

- Death literacy (understanding what dying looks like and what our options are)
- Family planning (discussing before a crisis occurs)
- Intentional death (choosing how we die instead of defaulting to hospital death)
- Community support in creating modern death rituals

We can take the best aspects of 1900 (death literacy, family involvement, planning) and combine them with the advancements of 2025 (medical progress, pain management, hospice). We can die better, but only if we're willing to talk about it. This book acts as a bridge from the denial of death in the present to a conscious acceptance of death in the past, updated for modern medicine and families. restores what was lost when death shifted into hospitals. The book shares what your great-grandmother understood instinctively: death is a natural part of life. It is inevitable. However, it can be approached with wisdom, preparation, and grace if we're brave enough to talk about it.

"Our great-grandparents knew how to die. Then death moved to the hospital, and we forgot. This book remembers."

CHAPTER 2:

The Cost of Silence

The key factor that often determines whether a death feels peaceful or traumatic is whether the family had talked about it beforehand.

Families who communicate openly understand what Dad wants, respect Mom's wishes, and ask questions before a crisis forces them to react. These families grieve, but they don't endure the additional trauma of uncertainty. They make decisions confidently because they're honoring wishes they already know.

Families who don't communicate often end up guessing, arguing, and making crisis decisions without guidance. They don't just mourn; they are traumatized by the experience of death itself. They carry guilt and regret that deepen their grief. This chapter shares stories of what happens when we fail to have the conversation. These are real stories (details changed to protect privacy, but circumstances remain accurate). These aren't rare cases; these are common scenarios that occur daily in hospitals, nursing homes, and ICUs across America.

I'm sharing these stories not to frighten you but to highlight what is at risk, as each of these tragic deaths could have been avoided with a simple conversation.

Story One: The Family Who Couldn't Agree

Tom's Story

When my father had his stroke, he was seventy-eight years old and in reasonably good health. He'd been gardening that morning and complained of a headache. He sat down and never got up again. The stroke was severe. The ER doctor said he'd survive, but he'd never walk again, never speak again, and might never recognize us. He needed a breathing tube immediately, then a feeding tube, and dialysis. The doctor asked: "Do you want us to do everything?" I had two siblings. We couldn't agree on anything. My sister Sarah said, "Dad's a fighter. He'd want us to try everything. We can't give up on him." My brother Mike said, "This isn't living. Dad loved golf, jokes, and being independent. He'd hate this. We should let him go."

I was caught in the middle: "I don't know what Dad wanted. He never told us." We fought. For three weeks, we argued in the ICU family waiting room while Dad lay in a medically induced coma surrounded by machines.

Sarah accused Mike of wanting Dad dead. Mike blamed Sarah for torturing Dad. I tried to mediate, but secretly agreed with Mike; this wasn't the life Dad would want.

Meanwhile, Dad's health worsened. He contracted pneumonia, then developed a pressure sore, then sepsis. The medical bills climbed: $15,000, $50,000, $100,000. Medicare covered most, but we paid out of pocket for the extras. Finally, after four weeks, Dad's heart stopped.

The ICU team asked, "Do you want us to resuscitate?"

Sarah screamed: "Yes! Do everything!"

Mike screamed: "No! Let him die in peace!"

I couldn't speak or move. I just stood there, paralyzed, as strangers pounded on my father's chest. They brought him back. His heart started again. He "lived" for another week before his kidneys completely failed, and the doctors said continuing was pointless. Even Sarah couldn't argue anymore.

Dad died on a Tuesday afternoon. None of us was there. Visiting hours had ended, and he died before we could get back.

The aftermath:

Sarah and Mike didn't speak for two years. I had nightmares for six months, seeing strangers pounding on Dad's chest while I stood frozen, unable to decide what he would have wanted. We all carried guilt: Sarah felt guilty for prolonging Dad's suffering. Mike felt guilty for not fighting harder to stop the treatment. I felt guilty for not having the courage to make a decision. The worst part? We never got to say goodbye. Dad was unconscious from the moment he had his stroke. We never told him we loved him. We never said it was okay to let go. We never asked him to forgive us for not knowing what he wanted.

What could have been different: If Dad had shared his wishes, if he'd said, "I don't want to be kept alive on machines if there's no hope of meaningful recovery," everything would have been different. We wouldn't have argued. We would have known what to do. We would have stopped treatment after the initial evaluation showed severe brain damage. We would have moved him to hospice, brought him home, if possible, surrounded him with family, music, and familiar comforts in his final days. We would have told him we loved him and said our goodbyes. Instead, we tortured him for five weeks because we didn't know what he wanted.

Story Two: The Medical Suffering No One Wanted

Linda's Story

My mother was eighty-six when she was diagnosed with stage 4 pancreatic cancer. Terminal. Inoperable. Maybe six months. The oncologist said, "We could try chemotherapy. It might extend her life by a few months. The side effects would be significant: nausea, fatigue, hair loss, and increased risk of infection. It's up to you." Mom looked at me. I looked at my sister. We looked at each other. Mom said weakly, "What should I do?" My sister said, "We should try everything. Maybe it'll work." I said, "But the side effects..." Mom said, "If you girls think I should try, I'll try." She didn't want chemotherapy. She was exhausted. She was ready to accept her death. But she didn't want to disappoint us. So, she underwent chemotherapy.

The first round made her extremely ill, and she vomited nonstop for three days. She lost fifteen pounds in a week and was so weak she could barely stand. The second round sent her to the hospital with neutropenic fever, a serious infection caused by chemo destroying her immune system. She spent a week in isolation. We could only visit in gowns and masks. She cried every day.

The third round left her with mouth sores so severe she couldn't eat or drink. She was readmitted for IV fluids and pain medication. After three months of chemotherapy, her cancer had grown. The treatment hadn't worked. She had suffered for nothing. The oncologist said, "We could try a different chemotherapy regimen..." This time, Mom said no. But it was already too late. She had spent three months being sick from treatment; three months she could have spent peacefully, at ease, surrounded by family. She died six weeks later. Her last three months on earth were filled with medical suffering she never wanted. At her funeral, I found a letter she had written but never sent.

Dear Girls,

I know you want me to fight, but I'm so tired. I don't want more treatment; I just want to be comfortable for whatever time I have left. I want to laugh with you, not vomit in a bucket. I want to hold my grandchildren, not lie in a hospital bed. But I can't tell you that because you'll think I'm giving up. So, I'll do what you want. I hope it doesn't take too long.

Love, Mom

I cried because she had endured chemotherapy for our sake, not for herself.

What could have been different:

If we had genuinely asked Mom what she wanted instead of assuming we knew, she would have told us: "No chemotherapy. I want quality, not quantity." If we had had that conversation before her cancer diagnosis, when she wasn't scared and sick, she would have been clear: "If I get terminal cancer, I don't want aggressive treatment. I want to be comfortable. I want to spend my last months at home with family, not in hospitals." We meant well. But our good intentions tortured her.

Story Three: The Financial Devastation

Robert's Story

My wife was diagnosed with ALS, Lou Gehrig's disease, at age fifty-seven. It's a progressive and fatal illness. There is no cure. The average life expectancy after diagnosis is 2 to 5 years. I was determined to care for her. We had been married for thirty-five years. I had promised to stand by her "in sickness and in health." I meant every word. I didn't realize what that promise would cost. During the first year, I managed. I learned how to use the feeding tube when she could no longer swallow. I learned transfers when she could no longer walk. I hired a part-time aide to assist with bathing.

The second year became more challenging. She needed 24/7 care. I hired full-time aides at $25 an hour, working around the clock, at a cost of about $18,000 per month. Medicare didn't cover these costs, and our savings began to dwindle.

In her third year, she required a ventilator.

The pulmonologist explained: "Two options. Hospice care, she'll pass when her breathing stops. Or ventilator support could keep her alive for years."

I asked, "What would you do?"

He said, "I can't tell you what to do. But I can tell you that ALS patients on long-term ventilators often become completely locked in, unable to move, unable to speak, unable to communicate, while remaining mentally alert. Quality of life becomes... questionable."

I asked my wife. She couldn't speak anymore, but she could still move her eyes. I held up two cards: "Hospice" and "Ventilator."

She looked at "Ventilator."

I believe she was trying to protect me, not to "give up' and to fight for her life. So, we chose the ventilator. The next two years were financially catastrophic. Round-the-clock nursing care costs us $30,000 a month. Specialized equipment added $10,000. Home modifications cost $50,000. Medications not covered by insurance cost $2,000 monthly. We drained our retirement savings, then our investments, mortgaged the house, and I borrowed money. After two years with the ventilator, my wife's eyes stopped moving. She was completely locked in. I couldn't tell if she was in pain, wanted to keep fighting, or regretted her decision. She died five years after her diagnosis. I was $400,000 in debt. The worst part? I found her advance directive in her desk drawer after she died. She had filled it out ten years earlier. It explicitly stated: "If I have a terminal illness and cannot communicate, I do NOT want to be kept alive on machines. I want comfort care only."

She had never told me it existed. I had never asked if she had one. If I had known that the document was available, she would have chosen hospice instead of the ventilator. She would have died two years earlier, peacefully and comfortably, without being trapped in her body for two years with no way to communicate.

And I wouldn't be bankrupt. I wouldn't have lost our house. I wouldn't be working at age seventy to pay off debt from medical care she never wanted.

Story Four: The Regret That Never Heals

Jennifer's Story

My father and I hadn't spoken for fifteen years. We'd had a falling out when I was twenty-five, over something trivial; my career choice disappointed him, and we exchanged harsh words, fueled by pride on both sides. Years of silence followed. When I was forty, I received the call: Dad had a massive heart attack. He was in the ICU, and I needed to come quickly. I flew across the country and sat beside his bedside. He was unconscious, on a ventilator, sedated. I waited for him to wake up so we could reconcile, so I could apologize, and he could apologize. We could have the conversation we should have had fifteen years earlier. But he never woke up. His brain had gone too long without oxygen, and the damage was permanent. After a week, the doctors said,

"He's not going to recover. You need to decide whether to keep him on life support."

I had to make the decision: me, his daughter, who hadn't spoken to him in fifteen years.

I had no idea what he would want. Did he have strong feelings about life support? Would he want to stay alive in a vegetative state? Would he want to donate his organs? Would he want a religious ceremony? I didn't know him anymore. I called his friends, coworkers, and neighbors. Asked everyone, "What would he want?" Nobody knew because no one talks about these things. I decided to withdraw life support. The doctors removed the breathing tube. Dad died two hours later. I held his hand. Told him I loved him. Apologized for the lost years. He never heard any of it. Ten years later, I'm still haunted: Did I make the right choice? Would he have wanted more time, even unconscious? Did he spend his last years thinking I hated him? Did he want to reconcile but was too proud to reach out? What would he have said if he'd woken up? I'll never know.

Contrast: What Happens When Families Do Talk

Before I show you the pattern in these stories, let me share one more, a different kind of story.

Margaret's Story

When my mother turned seventy-five, she gathered the family for Sunday dinner. After dessert, she said, "I want to talk about something uncomfortable: what happens when I'm dying."

We all tried to protest. She held up her hand.

Listen. I'm healthy now. I'm not dying today. But I will die eventually. And I don't want you kids guessing what I want. So, here's what I want," she pulled out papers she'd prepared.

I don't want to die in a hospital if I can help it. I want to come home and receive hospice care. I do NOT want CPR if my heart stops. I do

NOT want to be kept alive on machines. I do NOT want a feeding tube if I can't eat.

She looked each of us in the eye. "I know this is hard to hear. But I need you to promise you'll honor these wishes even if it's difficult. Even if you want to try 'just one more thing.' Promise me."

We promised. We cried. We asked questions. She answered them. We talked for two hours.

Then we moved on. Had coffee. Talked about grandkids and vacation plans. Life went on.

Five years later, Mom had a severe stroke. The ER doctor said she'd need a ventilator and feeding tube, but the prognosis was poor.

My brother and I looked at each other. We knew exactly what to do. "Mom has an advance directive," we said. "She doesn't want aggressive treatment. She wants comfort care only." We moved her to hospice that day and brought her home two days later. She was mostly unconscious but peaceful. We surrounded her with family, played her favorite music, and held her hands. We told her we loved her, thanked her for everything, and reassured her it was okay to let go. She died four days after her stroke, at home, surrounded by family—no tubes, no machines, no suffering. We grieved. God, we grieved. But we didn't feel guilty, uncertain, or regretful. We knew we had honored her wishes. We knew she had died the way she wanted. We knew we had done right by her. And that certainty made grief bearable.

This is what conversation makes possible.

Common Threads

These five stories are different: different circumstances, different outcomes, and different types of suffering. But the first four share common threads.

1. Crisis decisions without guidance. Not made thoughtfully with enough time to consider. Made in emergency rooms and ICU waiting rooms, with doctors asking, "What do you want us to do?" while nobody knew what the dying person wanted.

2. Good intentions, terrible outcomes. These families loved deeply and tried to do the right thing. However, without guidance, they made decisions driven by guilt, fear, and their own needs rather than the dying person's true wishes.

3. Trauma beyond death. These families didn't just grieve. They also carried guilt, regret, broken relationships, financial devastation, and unanswerable questions.

All of this was preventable. Not the deaths; those were inevitable. But the suffering, conflict, guilt, and trauma? All of it can be prevented through conversation.

The Real Cost Of Silence

When we don't talk about death before crisis strikes, the costs are devastating:

Medical costs:

- Unwanted aggressive treatment
- Extended ICU stays
- Procedures that prolong dying without improving living
- Average: $80,000+ per patient

Emotional costs:

- Family conflicts and broken relationships
- Guilt over decisions made
- Regret over words never spoken
- Trauma from witnessing preventable suffering.
- Unresolved complicated grief

Financial costs:

- Aggressive treatment not covered by insurance.

- 24/7 in-home care
- Lost work time for family caregivers
- Bankruptcy Due to Medical Debt
- Lost inheritances spent on unwanted care

Opportunity costs:

- Time spent in hospitals rather than at home
- Final months focused on treatment rather than connection.
- Conversations never took place because the patient was too sick.
- Goodbyes were never spoken because it happened too suddenly.
- Peace was never achieved because there was no time.

But the biggest cost is this: uncertainty.

Families who don't communicate beforehand often spend their lives wondering: "Did I make the right choice?" "Did they suffer because of my decision?" "Would they forgive me?" "Did they know I loved them?" These questions rarely have answers. That uncertainty worsens grief, making it feel longer, harder, and more painful.

The Choice Before You

You have a choice right now:

Option 1: Do nothing. Avoid the conversation. Wait until a crisis forces decisions. Choose one of the stories from earlier in this chapter: confusion, conflict, guilt, or uncertainty. Leave your family guessing about what you want. Guess what they want.

Option 2: Have the conversation. Uncomfortable? Yes. Necessary? Absolutely. Choose Margaret's story, clear wishes, honored decisions, peace amid grief. Give your family the gift of certainty. Accept that gift from them.

The difference between these two options is a conversation you've been avoiding.

"Silence doesn't protect us from death. It just ensures we're unprepared for it."

CHAPTER 3:

Why We Avoid the Conversation
(And Why Every Excuse Is Wrong)

—◆•●•◆—

The Most Dangerous Phrase In The English Language

We'll talk about it later.

I've heard this phrase countless times as a hospice nurse. We'll discuss it when Mom is feeling better. We'll have that conversation when Dad recovers from this setback. We'll talk about end-of-life wishes when the situation feels more urgent. Later. Always later. And then "later" becomes "too late." Mom never recovers; she declines and passes away before the talk. Dad doesn't bounce back from the setback; he has another stroke and loses the ability to speak. The urgency hits suddenly in an emergency room at 2 AM, when doctors need to make decisions, and no one knows what the patient wanted. "Later" is a lie we tell ourselves to avoid discomfort. And that lie costs everything.

In this chapter, we'll explore all the reasons you've avoided having this conversation. We'll understand why these reasons seem valid, then I'll explain why each one is actually wrong. This isn't about judging you; it's about showing how these beliefs can hurt you and those you care about.

EXCUSE #1: "Talking About It Makes It Happen Sooner"

Why you believe this:

Our culture has a long-standing superstition that speaking aloud gives words power. If you don't name something, it might not happen. Don't talk about death, and maybe it'll stay away. These beliefs go back thousands of years; ancient societies created taboos against saying the names of death gods, saying the word "death" openly, or acknowledging mortality. These superstitions have been passed down to us.

Why it feels true:

Correlation is mistaken for causation. You might know someone who discussed death and passed away soon after. Your mind creates a pattern: talking about death leads to death. Talking about death feels heavy. After such conversations, you're more aware of mortality, which increases anxiety and sadness. It seems like bringing up death has made it feel more imminent, not physically, but emotionally.

Why it's actually wrong:

Death is a biological process; cells age, organs fail, and bodies cease to function. Words don't alter this.

The truth:

- Talking about death doesn't cause it to happen faster.
- Avoiding discussions about death doesn't delay it.
- Death comes on its own schedule, completely indifferent to your conversations.

Here's what really happens: Talking about death gets you ready for its unavoidable arrival. That's all. That's everything.

The paradox: People who avoid talking about death because they fear it suffer the most when death arrives, unprepared, blindsided, and traumatized. Those who discuss death while healthy face it more peacefully because they're prepared.

Avoiding the conversation doesn't protect you from death. It guarantees you'll be unprepared for it.

EXCUSE #2: "It's Too Morbid/Depressing"

Why you believe this:

Our society has taught us to see death conversations as grim. We're encouraged to stay optimistic, hopeful, and focus on living instead of dying. Talking about death feels like dwelling on negativity. Plus, life is hard enough already. Why add more sadness?

Why it feels true:

Talking about death is often sad. Discussing losing loved ones hurts. After talking about end-of-life wishes, you might feel heavy, emotional, or even cry. Your brain thinks: this conversation made me sad, so it's bad, so I should avoid it.

Why it's actually wrong:

Morbid means "having an unhealthy obsession with death and disease." Having a thoughtful conversation about death wishes isn't morbid; it's pragmatic. The same level of morbidity as:

- Writing a will
- Buying life insurance
- Wearing a seatbelt
- Having a fire escape plan

None of these are morbid. They're sensible. Preparing for potential problems isn't dwelling on negativity; it's protecting yourself and those you love.

The truth:

The conversation itself isn't depressing. What's truly depressing is:

- Watching family members argue over what their dying loved one would have wanted.
- Making medical decisions driven by guilt rather than guidance
- Spending your last days enduring treatments you never wanted.

- Dying in a hospital instead of being at home
- Leaving your family behind causes trauma and regret.

That's depressing.

Talking about death while healthy feels awkward for an hour. Not talking about it causes trauma that lasts for years. Choose discomfort over trauma.

EXCUSE #3: "We Have Plenty of Time"

Why you believe this:

You're healthy. Your parents are healthy. No one is dying right now, so there's no urgent need for this conversation. You'll have it later, when it's more relevant.

Why it feels true:

Because most days, death feels far away. You wake up, go to work, and live your life. Death is an abstract, theoretical concept—something that happens to others. Your parents seem fine. Your spouse seems fine. You seem fine.

Why it's actually wrong:

Because death doesn't give advance warning, here's how it usually unfolds:

Monday: Everyone is healthy. No urgency to discuss death.

Tuesday: Mom experiences chest pain, goes to the ER, and has a heart attack.

Wednesday: Mom is in ICU, sedated and on a ventilator. The doctor asks, "What are her wishes?"

You respond: "I don't know. We never talked about it."

The shift from "we have plenty of time" to "we're out of time" happens within 48 hours.

The truth:

You might have decades, years, months, or just tomorrow. The only time you're sure of is now, today, this moment. When you say "we have plenty of time," you're avoiding discomfort by pretending it can wait. The real question isn't "Do we have time?" but "Why would you risk something this important?"

EXCUSE #4: "They'll Think I'm Giving Up"

Why it feels this way:

Our culture equates fighting with caring. "Keep fighting!" "Don't give up!" "Stay positive!" These phrases are everywhere. Planning for death seems like the opposite, like surrender, like betrayal.

Why it's wrong:

Fighting and planning aren't mutually exclusive. You can hope for the best and prepare for the worst.

Think about it: You wear a seatbelt, but that doesn't mean you're expecting to crash. You have home insurance, but that doesn't mean you think your house will burn down. You have a will, but that doesn't mean you're suicidal.

Preparing for bad outcomes while hoping for good ones isn't giving up. It's being smart.

The truth:

Not planning for death isn't a sign of hope; it's a sign of avoidance. And when death eventually occurs (because it always does), your lack of planning doesn't mean you fought harder; it just shows you're unprepared. The most caring thing you can do is hope your loved one recovers and make sure they're comfortable if they don't.

EXCUSE #5: "I Don't Want to Burden Them"

The fear:

Your children are busy. Your parents are fragile. Your spouse is stressed. Why add the burden of tough death conversations? You want to shield them from pain.

Why this backfires:

Not discussing death doesn't shield your family from the burden. It ensures they'll face an even heavier burden later, when it's much worse.

Small burden (having the conversation):

- One uncomfortable hour while everyone is healthy.
- Some tears, some discomfort.
- Then relief, clarity, and peace of mind.

Massive burden (not having the conversation):

- Making impossible medical decisions without guidance
- Family arguing over what you "would have wanted"
- Guilt over possibly making the wrong decision
- Financial ruin caused by unwanted treatments
- Years of regret and unanswered questions

What burden do you want to place on your family?

The truth:

The conversation feels uncomfortable for an hour. The silence creates trauma that can last for years. Avoiding the discussion doesn't protect your family; it only shields you from short-term discomfort while putting their long-term well-being at risk. This isn't love. It's avoidance pretending to be love.

EXCUSE #6: "They'll Think I Don't Love Them"

The fear:

If you tell your mother, "I don't want CPR if my heart stops," she might think you don't value life. If you ask your father, "What do you want if you have a massive stroke?" he might think you're trying to get rid of him. Our culture teaches that loving someone means doing everything to keep them alive. So, planning for death feels like its opposite, not loving enough.

The truth:

Love isn't about denying death. Love is about honoring wishes. True love says: I love you so much that I want to understand what YOU want; not what I want for you, not what doctors suggest, and not what society expects. I want to honor your wishes because respecting your autonomy is part of respecting love for you.

The bottom line:

Avoiding death conversations doesn't mean more love. It reflects a preference for your own comfort rather than their peace of mind. Having the conversation demonstrates that I love you enough to face difficult topics, respect your wishes even if they differ from mine, and ensure your death aligns with your values.

EXCUSE #7: "It's Too Uncomfortable"

The reality:

Yes, this conversation is uncomfortable. Death is a heavy topic. We stumble over words. We cry. We laugh nervously. We change the subject. Discomfort is real. But what's even more uncomfortable: standing in an ICU at 2 AM, trying to decide whether to pull the plug on your father while having no idea what he'd want; watching your mother suffer through chemotherapy she never wanted because you were too uncomfortable to ask; spending your final weeks in a hospital you hate because your family assumed you'd want "everything done."

The choice:

The conversation is uncomfortable for an hour, but the alternative can be traumatic for years. Choose discomfort over trauma.

EXCUSE #8: "I Don't Know What to Say"

This statement accurately reflects current ability.

Most people don't know how to start this conversation. We aren't taught this. There's no class in school called "How to Discuss Death with Your Family." We lack models because our parents didn't talk about it, and their parents didn't either.

But "I don't know how" is different from "I can't."

You didn't know how to change a diaper until you had a baby; then you learned. You didn't know how to file taxes until you had to; then you learned. You don't know how to talk about death, but you can learn.

The truth is:

The next part of this book provides exactly what you need: the tools, scripts, and specific words to use. "I don't know how" is a valid statement of current ability, but it is not a valid reason for doing nothing.

The Underlying Fear Beneath All Excuses

All of these excuses come down to the same fundamental fear:

Acknowledging death makes it real, and I don't want it to be.

This is the human condition. We know intellectually that we'll die, but emotionally, we believe we're the exception. Death happens to others, not to us or our loved ones. This phenomenon is called "mortality salience," the psychological discomfort we experience when confronted with our own mortality. It's normal. It's human. It's uncomfortable. And it's precisely why we need to talk about it.

Because death doesn't care about your discomfort. Death doesn't wait until you're ready. Death doesn't only come after you've had the conversation. Death comes on its own schedule. And your only choice is whether you'll be prepared.

The Real Question

The question isn't: "Is this conversation uncomfortable?" Obviously, it's uncomfortable. The real question is: "Is my discomfort more important than my family's future trauma?" Because those are the stakes.

Your options:

Option A: Have one uncomfortable hour-long conversation while everyone is healthy.

- Discomfort Level: Medium
- Duration: 1 hour
- Outcome: Clear understanding, peace of mind, and a prepared family

Option B: Steer clear of the conversation to prevent discomfort.

- Discomfort Level: Zero (currently)
- Duration: Until a crisis occurs
- Outcome: Family confusion, guilt, trauma, and regret that last for years or decades.

The math is simple. One hour of discomfort versus years of trauma. You're opting for trauma to dodge discomfort.

"Your silence is a burden you carry, while your voice is a gift you offer today".

CHAPTER 4:

The Birth/Death Paradox:
Why We Plan for One but Not the Other

———— ◆●◆●◆ ————

Two Certainties, Two Responses

Two events are absolutely certain in human life: birth and death. Every person who has ever existed has been born. Every person will eventually die. These are the two certainties. Now, let me show you how we respond to these unavoidable realities.

How We Plan For Birth

Nine months before birth: Pregnancy test positive. Planning begins within hours.

Months 1-2:

- Schedule prenatal checkups
- Research obstetricians
- Take prenatal vitamins.
- Tell family and friends.

Months 3-4:

- Register for childbirth classes
- Visit hospitals or birthing centers
- Research pediatricians.
- Begin preparing the baby's room.
- Read books about pregnancy and newborn care.

Months 5-6:

Write birth plan:

- o Natural birth or epidural?
- o Hospital, birthing center, or home?
- o Who will be present in the delivery room?
- o What interventions are acceptable or not?
- o What happens if complications occur?
    - Register for baby items.
    - Attend a baby shower
    - Pack your hospital bag.

Months 7-8:

- Finalize the birth plan.
- Discuss your plan with your doctor or midwife.
- Tour the hospital's labor and delivery department.
- Complete pre-registration for hospital
- Install car seat.
- Stock up on supplies for a newborn

Month 9:

Have an in-depth discussion with the birthing partner about:

- When to go to the hospital
- What to do if labor begins suddenly
- Who to contact
- What you want and don't want during labor
- Pain management preferences
- Your fears and hopes

Everything is prepared. When labor begins, everyone is aware of the plan. Everyone understands their role. The mother's wishes are recorded and respected. Decisions are made based on previously discussed preferences, not out of panic.

After birth:

- Comprehensive postpartum recovery plan
- Feeding plans organized
- Scheduled parental leave
- Support system established
- Follow-up appointments scheduled

Total for birth planning:

- Planning time: Nine months of dedicated effort
- Conversations: Dozens
- Documentation: Birth plan, hospital pre-registration, insurance paperwork, pediatrician chosen
- Cultural support: Whole industry (birthing classes, books, apps, support groups)
- Social acceptance: Obsessing over birth planning is perfectly normal.

How We "Plan" For Death

Decades before death: nothing.

Years before death: Possibly a vague feeling that we should write a will "someday."

Months before death: Still nothing unless there's a diagnosis. Even then, often denial.

Weeks before death: Possibly some emergency conversations if the person remains conscious, but usually not.

Days before death: Panic. Crisis. Doctors ask, "What do you want us to do?" Family has no idea.

When death approaches:

- Nobody knows the plan (there isn't one).
- Nobody understands their role

- The wishes of the person who is dying are unknown.
- Decisions motivated by panic, guilt, and confusion

After death:

- Family discovers (or fails to discover) what the person wanted—too late.
- Regret, guilt, and uncertainty
- Family conflict

Total for death planning:

- Planning time: Usually none.
- Conversations: Usually none.
- Documentation: Sometimes a will, rarely advance directives, seldom a comprehensive death plan.
- Cultural support: None; actively discouraged ("Don't be morbid!").
- Social acceptance: Perceived as strange, morbid, or pessimistic.

The Paradox

We spend nine months carefully planning for an event (birth) that:

- Occurs once or only a few times in a lifetime
- We have some influence over
- Modern medicine has become incredibly safe.
- Usually goes smoothly.
- Leads to happiness

We spend no time planning for an event (death) that::

- Happens to all of us, guaranteed.
- Our control over is limited.
- Medicine cannot prevent, only delay.
- Often involves tough decisions
- Results in grief compounded by trauma if unplanned.

This doesn't make sense. Logically, we should plan MORE for death than for birth, not less.

Why The Paradox Exists

Historical reasons:

For most of human history, both birth and death occurred at home. Both were family events, familiar and communal. Then medicine changed everything. Birth was medicalized, moved to hospitals, overseen by doctors, but eventually came full circle. Today, we have birth plans, midwives, birthing centers, and home births. We've reclaimed birth planning.

Death was also medicalized, moved to hospitals, and managed by doctors, and it mostly stayed there. We haven't reclaimed death planning yet. It is still viewed as medical territory, not personal or family space.

Cultural reasons:

- We celebrate life. We fear death.
- Talking about birth is socially acceptable. Discussing death is taboo.
- Birth planning is regarded as responsible, while death planning is viewed as morbid.
- Birth classes are common. Death classes aren't available (except in hospice, when it's too late).

Psychological reasons:

- Birth happens to other people (the baby). Death happens to us.
- Birth feels like a new beginning. Death feels like a final ending.
- Birth is filled with hope. Death is filled with fear.
- We tend to make plans for things we're excited about, but avoid planning for things we fear.

But here's what all these reasons overlook: Both birth and death greatly benefit from planning.

What If We Planned For Death As We Plan For Birth?

Imagine this alternative reality:

Ages 20-30: Early Death Education

Just as people learn about pregnancy and childbirth, they also learn about aging and dying. Death literacy becomes normal:

- What defines a good death versus a bad death?
- What are your choices at the end of life?
- What are hospice and palliative care?
- What are advance directives?

Ages 30-40: First Death Conversations

Just as couples discuss if and when to have children, families talk about death wishes.

Sunday dinner conversations include:

- What would you want if you were in a vegetative state?
- Have you thought about DNR orders?
- Would you prefer to die at home or in a facility?

As normal as talking about where you want your kids to go to college.

Ages 40-50: Death Planning

Just as parents plan for their children's future, adults plan for their own death. They:

- Write living wills.
- Designate a healthcare power of attorney

Document wishes regarding life support, feeding tubes, CPR, quality of life benchmarks, preferred place of death, sources of comfort, and designated individuals to be present.

Ages 50-60: Regular Updates

Just as you update your will when circumstances change, you should also regularly update your death wishes. After major life events:

- Divorce/remarriage → Update healthcare proxy
- Diagnosis → Refine wishes based on condition
- Child becomes adult → Discuss wishes with them
- Parent dies → Reflect, and adjust own plans

Ages 60-70: Detailed Planning

Just as people plan their retirement in detail, they also plan their end-of-life in detail. Conversations often include specific DNR preferences, hospice versus hospital choices, pain management philosophies, religious wishes, legacy projects, funeral preferences, and final letters written while healthy.

Ages 70+: Maintenance & Readiness

Just as older adults regularly update estate documents, they also keep their death plans current.

Regular family meetings:

- Has anything about your wishes changed?
- Do you still want X to serve as your healthcare proxy?
- Is there anything you want to tell us while you still can?

When serious illness arrives:

Family already knows:

- What the person desires and avoids
- Who makes decisions?

- What quality of life means to them
- What fears do they have, and what brings them peace?

Decisions are guided by documented wishes, not panic. When death nears, everyone is prepared, and the plan is put into action. Wishes are respected. Death remains sad, but it is no longer traumatic.

What This Looks Like: Real Stories

The Anderson Family

Every Thanksgiving, after dinner, the Anderson family has what they call "the conversation."

It started when the matriarch, Helen (now 72), turned 50. She said, "Life is good. But we all know we won't live forever. Let's make sure we're all on the same page about what we want."

At first, her adult children felt uneasy. But Helen persisted. Every year, she would ask: Have anyone's wishes changed? Do you understand what I want? Have you thought about what you want?

By the fifth year, it felt normal, routine, like talking about holiday plans.

When Helen was diagnosed with aggressive breast cancer at 68, everything was already in place.

- Her wishes are documented.
- Her children knew she preferred quality rather than quantity.
- She'd already decided: if treatment had less than a 30% chance of significantly extending her life, she'd choose hospice over chemo.
- She had already told them where she wanted to die (at home).
- She had already written letters to all her grandchildren.
- She had already planned her funeral.

When the oncologist said, "The cancer is aggressive. Chemo might give you six more months, but they'll be hard months," Helen responded immediately: "Then I choose hospice. I choose home. I choose quality." Her children didn't argue or feel guilty; they supported her decision because they knew it was her choice, not made in panic but confirmed over the years. Helen lived six months on hospice, comfortable, precious months, spent with grandchildren, finishing legacy projects, and saying everything she wanted to say. She died at home, surrounded by family, exactly as she'd planned. At her funeral, her daughter said, "Mom gave us the greatest gift: she told us what she wanted. We didn't have to guess. We didn't have to fight. We didn't have to carry guilt. We just had to honor her wishes. And that made the unbearable bearable."

This is what planning makes possible.

The Patel Family

Raj and Anjali Patel are in their early 40s with two young children. After Raj's father died suddenly from a heart attack, leaving the family in chaos with no guidance, Raj decided, "This won't happen to my family."

They took these steps:

1. Had "the conversation" with each other:

- Created living wills.
- Designated healthcare proxies
- Discussed specific scenarios (vegetative state: consider withdrawal; terminal cancer: prioritize quality of life over longevity; Alzheimer's: hospice when appropriate, avoid feeding tubes).

2. Documented everything:

- Legal documents filed
- Copies to healthcare proxies
- Doctor notified.
- Documents stored safely at home and in cloud storage

3. Update annually:

- Every anniversary, they review
- Takes about 30 minutes.
- Usually no changes, but peace of mind is renewed.

4. Talked to their parents:

- Assisted both families in creating advance directives.
- Now everyone knows everyone's wishes.

5. Age-appropriately discussed with their children:

- At age 6: "If something happens to Mommy or Daddy, you'll live with Aunt Sarah"
- Age 10: "When people get very old or very sick, their bodies stop working. It's sad but natural."
- Age 14: "Let's discuss what Grandma wants if she becomes too ill to tell us."

The result:

If tragedy strikes the Patel family, everyone knows what to do. No confusion. No conflict. No guessing. Paradoxically, this planning doesn't cause them anxiety; it brings them peace. They live fully because they've prepared for death. This is what planning enables.

Completing The Circle

Think of life as a circle; a practical, human journey from start to finish.

The circle begins with birth. We plan carefully, prepare, and celebrate. We create safety and structure around this transition. Baby showers, birth plans, and hospital tours are all culturally normal, socially celebrated, and practically supported.

The circle goes on through life. We plan for milestones: education, career, marriage, and children. We set goals. We prepare. We openly discuss what we want our lives to become.

The circle should end with death, but this is where we stop planning; where preparation becomes taboo. The circle breaks precisely when families need it most.

When the circle is incomplete:

- Shock at the approach of death (even when expected)
- Panic instead of preparation
- Guessing rather than knowing
- Fighting rather than unity
- Trauma over peace

When the circle is complete:

- Death planning occurs alongside birth planning.
- Families discuss death as naturally as they discuss birth.
- Children acquire death literacy in the same way they learn about birth.
- End-of-life wishes are discussed as openly as birth plans.
- Dying is honored with the same preparation as being born.

The circle completes a family at a time. You don't need to wait for cultural change; you can start in your family today. Reading this book is already a step toward breaking the silence. By having the conversation, you normalize death planning. By establishing an Annual Review, you create a tradition your children will carry on. The circle is completed one family at a time. Your family could be next.

"We prepare for birth because we celebrate it. We should prepare for death because we honor it. Both are sacred. Both deserve preparation".

PART TWO:

THE CONVERSATION

How to start the most important conversation of your life

CHAPTER 5:

Preparing for the Conversation

—————————————◆●◆●◆————————————

The Moment Before

Rachel sat in her car outside her parents' house, her heart pounding. She had driven two hours for "the conversation." She was ready, but she hesitated to open the door. What if they think I'm trying to get rid of them? What if I say the wrong thing? Her phone buzzed: "Are you coming in? Pot roast is getting cold." She took a deep breath, opened the door, and three hours later, returned to her car with her parents' completed advance directives and tears; the good kind. Her mother had said, "Thank you for being brave enough to ask. We've wanted to talk but didn't know how." The hardest part was opening the car door.

Preparing Yourself

Get Clear on Your "Why"

Before this conversation, be very clear about why you're doing it. Not just "I should," but your true, personal reason.

Good reasons:

- I love them and prefer not to guess.
- I saw my aunt's family break apart because of this.
- Making decisions without guidance traumatized me.

Your "why" is your anchor when conversations get tough.

Examine Your Fears

Write down all your fears. Then face each one.
Fear: "They'll think I want them dead."
Reality: People who love you don't assume the worst.

Fear: "I'll say the wrong thing."

Reality: Perfect words don't exist. Authenticity is enough.

Fear: "This will ruin our relationship."

Reality: Avoiding tough conversations damages relationships. Facing them builds intimacy.

Most fears are catastrophizing. The actual conversation is rarely as bad as you imagine.

Release the Need for Perfect

There's no perfect way to have this talk. You'll stumble, search for words, maybe cry. It will be messy.

That's okay. What matters isn't perfect words, but showing up with love and courage.

Prepare for Emotions

Emotions that might show up:

For you: anxiety, sadness, relief, guilt, love. For them: fear, sadness, anger, resistance, gratitude. All are normal. Hold space for emotions. Don't try to suppress them.

Practice saying: "This is hard. It's okay to feel [sad/scared/angry]."

Am I Ready?

Before scheduling, ask yourself:

□ Do I understand WHY this matters (emotionally, not just intellectually)?
□ Have I examined my fears?
□ Can I stay calm if they get upset?
□ Am I doing this out of love, not obligation?
□ Can I accept that they might not be ready yet?

Mostly, yes? You're ready.

The Logistics
When to Have It

Best time: When everyone is healthy, calm, and has time together.

Good triggers:

- After a funeral, everyone's thinking about mortality.
- Milestone birthdays (60th, 70th, 75th)
- During holidays when families are already gathered
- Following a health scare
- Honestly, just a typical Sunday dinner. Sometimes the best moment is right now.

Times to avoid:

- During a crisis
- When someone is very ill
- During family conflicts
- When emotions are already running high

Where to Have It

Good locations:

- Their home (cozy, familiar)
- Your home (where you control the environment)
- During a walk (walking side-by-side feels easier)
- Neutral location (quiet restaurant, park)

Bad locations:

- Party or gathering.
- In a car.
- By text or email
- In a hospital.

Set up the space:

- Privacy (no TV, no interruptions)
- Comfort (good seating)
- Time (allow 1-2 hours)
- Materials (paper and pen ready)

How to Bring It Up

Three strong approaches:

1. Direct:
"I want to talk about something important. Can we discuss end-of-life wishes?"

2. Story-triggered:
"After [event], I realized I don't know what you'd want. Can we talk?"

3. Vulnerability:
"I've been thinking about mortality. I want to know your wishes."

The formula that works:

- Acknowledge difficulty: "This isn't easy..."
- State intention: "...but I want to know your wishes..."
- Express love: "...because you matter to me."
- Request permission: "Can we talk?"

Give Warning

Don't ambush people.

Say something like:
"I'd like to talk about end-of-life wishes—not because anyone's dying, but because I want to know. Can we set aside time this week?"

This gives them:

- Time to prepare
- Control over timing
- Sense of what's coming

What to Bring

Notebook and pen
Blank advance directive forms
Tissues
Water
Your "why" (mental preparation)
Questions to ask
Patience
Compassion

The Mindset

The Energy You Bring

Come with:

- Love (not fear)
- Curiosity (not assumptions)
- Respect (not pity)
- Openness (not agenda)
- Calmness (not anxiety)

Your energy sets the tone.

The Goal

This conversation is NOT about:

- Filling out all forms today.
- Having a perfect conversation.
- Convincing them of anything.

This conversation IS about:

- Beginning the conversation
- Hearing what they want
- Fostering safety for future discussions
- Documenting what you learn

Progress over perfection.

Core Principles

1. **About THEM, not you:** Listen to THEIR wishes, not your opinions.
2. **Honor autonomy:** Even if you disagree, THEIR wishes matter.
3. **Remain curious:** Don't jump to conclusions. Ask questions. Really listen.
4. **Create a safe environment:** No wrong answers.
5. **Be patient:** it may take several conversations.

Handling Different Outcomes

If It Goes Badly - "Badly" might refer to refusal, anger, shutdown, or accusations.

What to do: Don't take it personally. Their resistance stems from fear, not you.

Acknowledge: "I see this is hard."

Clarify: "I'm not trying to push you toward anything."

Offer space: "We don't have to talk today."

Leave the door open: "When you're ready, I'm here."

Try again later using a different approach and timing. Accept that there are limitations: some people won't be ready. You did your best.

If It Goes Well - Well, "might" suggests relief, openness, sharing, and closeness.

What to do: Show appreciation: "Thank you for trusting me."

Document everything: Take notes immediately.

Follow through: Do what you said you'd do.

Check in regularly: "Has anything changed?"

Respect their trust: Never share without permission.

Common Obstacles & Responses

I'm not ready.
→ "I understand. But can we try? I care too much to drop this."

Why now? Am I dying? → "Not at all! I'm asking BECAUSE you're healthy."

I don't want to burden you.
→ "Not knowing is the burden. This conversation is a gift."

I'm fine with whatever you decide.
→ "I appreciate your trust, but I need to know what YOU want."

Let's not be morbid.
→ "This isn't morbid, it's practical. Like having a will."

They cry:
→ [Hand tissues] "It's okay to cry. Take your time." [Silence. Continue when ready.]

"Courage isn't the absence of fear. It's opening the car door anyway".

CHAPTER 6:

Having the Conversation:
Scripts for Every Relationship

───────── ◆◗●◗◆ ─────────

The Conversations That Change Everything

Three families. Three conversations. Three different relationships.

Maria and her 72-year-old mother: "Mom, I need to talk to you about something. I want to know what you'd want if you got very sick." Her mother paused mid-dish. "Oh. That." "Yes. That." "I've been hoping you'd ask. I've been too scared to bring it up."

David and Jennifer, married for 15 years, on a hike: "If something happened to me, would you know what I'd want?" David stopped walking. "What do you mean? Are you sick?" "No. But we've never talked about it. And I realized, we should."

Eleanor and her three adult children: "I have something important to discuss. I'm healthy. Nothing's wrong. But I want to tell you what I want when I'm dying." Daughter Sarah protested, "Mom, don't talk like that." Eleanor raised her hand. "Listen. I'm going to die someday. And I don't want you three fighting or carrying guilt. So, I'm going to tell you." Three different dynamics. Same essential conversation.

This chapter gives you the tools for all of them.

Talking To Your Parents

Why Parent Conversations Are Different

Power dynamics are complex. They raised you, and it's hard for them to see you as capable of having this discussion. You're acknowledging that they'll die (and that you will too). Cultural messaging says children shouldn't discuss their parents' death. But this conversation is one of the most loving things you can do.

Special Considerations

If you have siblings:

- Best: Have a conversation together (everyone hears the same thing)
- Reality: Often one child bears most of the burden.
- Solution: Record everything and share with siblings right away

Which parent to talk to first:

- Best: Both together (they decide together)
- Alternative: Talk to a more open parent first; they might bring the other along.

Cultural and religious considerations:
Respect the culture AND speak gently: "I know in our culture we don't talk about this. But I love you too much not to know what you want."

How to Start: Three Approaches

1. DIRECT
"I want to talk about something important. It's about end-of-life wishes. I know it's not easy, but I need to know what you'd want if something happened."

2. STORY-TRIGGERED
"After [funeral/health scare], I realized I don't know what you'd want. Seeing what their family went through made me realize how messy things get without a plan. Can we talk?"

3. VULNERABILITY
I've been concerned about what might happen if you got sick and I didn't know what you'd want. Can we talk about that?

Handling Common Resistance

I'm not ready to talk about this.
→ "I know this is scary, but I'm more scared of not knowing. Can we just get started?"

Why are you bringing this up? Am I dying?
→ "No! I'm bringing it up BECAUSE you're healthy. This is the best time, when there's no crisis."

I trust you kids to decide.
→ "I appreciate your trust. But I don't want to guess. What would YOU want?"

Let's talk about this later.
→ "When later? Can we put it on the calendar? This matters too much to keep postponing."

They start crying:
→ [Hand tissues] "It's okay to cry. Take your time. This is hard." [Wait. Then continue when ready.]

What to Ask Your Parents

Treatment philosophy:
"If you had a terminal illness with no hope of recovery, would you prefer aggressive treatment or comfort care?"

Specific scenarios:

- What if you experienced a severe stroke and ended up in a vegetative state?
- What if you had dementia and couldn't recognize us?
- If your heart stopped, would you want CPR?

Location and presence:
"Where would you want to be? Who do you want with you?"

Healthcare proxy:
"Who do you want making decisions if you can't? Primary person? Backup?"

Talking To Your Spouse/Partner

Why Partner Conversations Are Different

This is mutual planning. You both share AND listen. You're likely each other's healthcare proxies. You'll probably make decisions for one another. You're acknowledging that one of you will likely watch the other die. But you chose this person. You trust them. You've navigated tough situations together. This conversation deepens your bond.

How to Start: Three Approaches

1. DIRECT
I want to discuss end-of-life wishes, both yours and mine. We've never talked about this, and I believe we should.

2. TRIGGERED
"After [event], I've been thinking, if something happened to one of us, would the other know what we wanted?"

3. VULNERABLE
"I love you so much, and the thought of losing you terrifies me. But what terrifies me more is not knowing what you'd want."

The Framework: Mutual Sharing

This isn't an interrogation. It's mutual vulnerability.

Structure:

1. Set the stage: "This might be hard. Let's be honest and loving."
2. Take turns sharing (10-15 minutes each)
3. Ask clarifying questions
4. Find alignment and differences

5. Document together

Key Questions to Explore Together

Quality of Life: "What makes life worth living to you? What would make it not worth living?"

Treatment philosophy: "If terminal illness with maybe 6 months left, aggressive treatment or comfort care?"

Specific scenarios: Walk through sudden accidents, vegetative states, cancer with treatment options, slow decline, and heart-stopping situations.

Location and presence: "Where do you want to be? Who's with you?"

Your role: "What do you need from me as you're dying?"

After death: "What do you want me to know about after you die?" (Permission to move on? How to handle belongings? Messages for kids?)

Handling Disagreements

Different treatment philosophies: 'We want different things. That's okay. I'll honor what YOU want for yourself." Plan separately. Respect autonomy.

Who should be present: Explore the why, find a compromise, and ensure the dying person has the final say.

Moving on after death: 'I can't promise what I'll do 5 years after you die. But I can promise I'll always love you."

Special Scenarios

Terminal illness (death imminent, not theoretical): "Are there things you want to do, see, or say before you die? What would bring you peace?"

Second marriage/blended family: Clearly establish authority. Document to avoid conflicts.

Unmarried partners: CRITICAL: Legal healthcare power of attorney is essential! Without marriage, you may have NO legal right to make decisions.

LGBTQ+ couples: Extra protections necessary—secure airtight legal documents, keep multiple copies with trusted friends, and find identified LGBTQ+-friendly healthcare providers.

Talking To Your Adult Children (About Your Wishes)

Why This Conversation Is Different

The roles are reversed. You're preparing them for YOUR death. You're vulnerable to mortality. You hold authority, but they'll have power when you can't decide. You're asking them to imagine life without you. But this is one of the most loving things you can do as a parent.

Special Considerations

Multiple children: Best to tell them all together (everyone hears the same thing, no "broken telephone").

One child as healthcare proxy:
"I've chosen [name] because [reason]. I need you all to support them." Document this clearly to prevent resentment.

Estranged children: Consider whether they need to know and if they might try to override this. Legal documents prevent it.

Only child: Extra burden. Name backup proxy. Acknowledge: "This is a lot to put on you alone."

How to Start: Three Approaches

1. DIRECT
"I want to talk about something important. I'm healthy, but I won't be forever. I want to tell you what I want when I'm dying."

2. TRIGGERED
"After [funeral/health scare], I realized I've never told you what I'd want."

3. GIFT FRAMING
"I want to give you a gift: the gift of knowing my wishes so you won't have to guess."

What to Tell Them

Be very clear. This is not the time to shield them from sad feelings.

Your treatment philosophy:
"If I have a terminal illness with no hope of recovery, I do NOT want aggressive treatment. I want comfort care only."

OR: "I want to try treatment if there's at least a 20% chance of meaningful recovery."

Specific scenarios:

- If I have a massive stroke and remain in a vegetative state, pull the plug after [timeframe].
- If I have dementia and can no longer recognize you, I do NOT want a feeding tube. Let me die naturally.
- If my heart stops: Do NOT do CPR if I'm over 80 or have a terminal illness.

BE SPECIFIC. Vague information isn't helpful when they're in the ICU at 2 AM.

Location: "I want to die at home if possible."

Who present: "I want all of you there" OR "just [name]" OR "I don't want you watching me die."

What matters most: "Being pain-free is most important." "Being at home matters more than extra time."

Your fears:

- "I'm most afraid of dying in pain." → They'll prioritize pain management
- "I'm afraid of dying alone." → They'll make sure someone's always there

Healthcare proxy: "[Name], I'm naming you. Here's why. [To siblings:] Support your sister. Her decision is final."

After you die: "Don't rush grief. Sell the house if keeping it is too hard. Use life insurance for [purpose]."

Handling Their Responses

Don't talk like that, Mom/Dad!
→ "I know this is hard. But I'm going to die someday. I love you too much to leave you guessing."

You're not dying anytime soon!
→ "I hope you're right. But hope isn't a plan. I need to tell you while I can."

I can't handle this conversation.
→ "I understand it's overwhelming. But I need you to handle it. If something happens and you don't know my wishes, that will be much harder."

What if I make the wrong decision?

→ "There is no wrong decision if you're honoring my wishes. I'm telling you what I want. Your job is to follow through."

Crying (can't speak):

→ [Hand tissue] "I know. Take your time. This is hard because you love me." [Wait. Continue when ready.]

After Any Conversation

Immediate steps:

- Thank them.
- Record everything right away.
- Confirm understanding: "Let me make sure I heard correctly..."
- Complete advance directives.
- Distribute copies to everyone who needs them.

Follow-up:

- Give copies to their doctor.
- Store documents correctly.
- Schedule annual review.

Ongoing:

- Review annually
- Update following health changes
- Keep the conversation open.

Universal Principles

Before any conversation:

- Clarify your "why."
- Face your fears (often just catastrophizing)
- Let go of perfectionism.

During the conversation:

- Come from love, not fear
- Stay curious and don't make assumptions.
- Create a safe environment (no wrong answers).
- Be patient; it may require several conversations.

Your goal: Start the conversation. Don't try to do everything perfectly today.

The Deeper Gift

These conversations do more than just document wishes.

Parent conversations: Free them from uncertainty, prevent family conflict, and honor their autonomy.

Partner conversations: Deepen intimacy, build trust, face mortality together, and strengthen your partnership.

Children conversations: Teach courage, model death wisdom, give them clarity, and protect them from guilt.

All of these: Transform death from a taboo into something normal, change your family culture, and complete the circle.

"Three conversations. Three relationships. One message: I love you enough to have this hard talk".

CHAPTER 7:

The Essential Questions: What to Ask

◆●◆

The Power Of The Right Question

When Dr. Martinez's father had a massive heart attack, the ER doctor asked, "Do you want us to intubate?" Dr. Martinez, despite being a physician herself, froze. "I... I don't know." "What would your father want?" "I don't know. We never talked about it." They intubated. Her father survived initially but never regained consciousness. After three weeks of organ failure and suffering, he died in the ICU. Years later, Dr. Martinez learned from an old friend, "Your dad always said he never wanted to be kept alive on machines." One question she never asked cost her father the death he wanted. This chapter provides those questions.

Why Specific Questions Matter

General statements are unhelpful during a crisis:

"I want everything done." → What's everything? For how long? "I don't want to suffer." → What level of suffering is acceptable? "Whatever you think is best." → That's not helpful when deciding at 2 AM.

Specific questions get specific answers:

"If your heart stops, do you want CPR?" → Clear yes/no "Would you want a feeding tube if you had advanced dementia?" → Clear scenario, clear answer

This chapter is your menu. Choose what's relevant.

The Essential Questions

1. Quality Of Life

"What makes life worth living for you?"
"What would make life NOT worth living anymore?"
"How important is independence to you?"
"How important is staying mentally sharp?" (For many, losing their mind is worse than losing their body)
"How do you feel about pain versus being alert?" (Pain-free but drowsy vs. alert with some pain?)

2. Treatment Preferences

Philosophy:
"If you had a terminal illness with no hope of recovery, would you prefer aggressive treatment to prolong life or comfort care focused on quality?"

CPR:
"If your heart stopped, would you want CPR?"
(Explain: Often breaks ribs, low success rates, risk of brain damage)
"Would your answer change if you were 90? If you had terminal cancer?"

Ventilator:
"If you couldn't breathe on your own, would you want a breathing machine?"

- Short-term (days/weeks) while recovering?
- Long-term (months/permanent) if chronic condition?
- Indefinitely if vegetative state?

Feeding Tube:
"If you couldn't eat or drink, would you want a feeding tube?"

- Temporary (stroke recovery)?
- Permanent (advanced dementia)?

Dialysis:
"If your kidneys failed, would you want dialysis?"

- Temporary while recovering?
- What would you do long-term if you had terminal cancer?

Antibiotics:
"If you developed pneumonia, would you want antibiotics?"

- If you had advanced dementia?
- If you were in hospice with terminal cancer?

3. Location And Presence

Where would you want to be when you're dying? (Home, hospital, hospice facility, nursing home?)

What if going home isn't medically feasible?

Who do you want with you? (Everyone, immediate family, just one person, nobody?)

Do you want young children or grandchildren to see you very sick? (Say goodbye? Or be remembered as you were?)

4. Values And Priorities

Rank these by importance:

- Length of life
- Quality of life
- Independence
- Mental clarity
- Being at home
- Minimal suffering
- Time with family
- Following religious beliefs

Would you prefer quantity over quality? Three comfortable months versus six months of significant suffering?

What does 'being a burden' mean to you? (Financial? Physical care? Emotional? Time?)

5. Fears And Concerns

What worries you the most about dying?

(Common: pain, being alone, losing dignity, losing your mind, becoming a burden)

What steps can I take to prevent or deal with that fear?

Is there anything you'd need to do, say, or resolve before you can die peacefully? (Reconcile with someone? Attend a specific event? Finish a project?)

6. Spiritual And Religious

Do your religious or spiritual beliefs influence what you'd want for end-of-life care? (Specific rituals? Certain treatments prohibited or required?)

What do you believe occurs after death? (Not to debate, but to understand what brings peace)

Is there a religious leader you'd like us to contact? (Name, contact info, best time to call)

Are there particular religious or cultural rituals that are important to you? (Last rites, prayers, facing a specific direction, etc.)

7. Practical And Legal

Who do you want to make medical decisions if you're unable to? (Primary person? Backup? Does this person know you're choosing them?)

Would you like a DNR (Do Not Resuscitate) order? (Clarifies no CPR, but other care continues)

Do you want to be an organ donor? (All organs? Specific ones only? For transplant or research?)

Are there financial limits to treatment you want us to respect? (Would you want expensive treatment if it bankrupted the family?)

8. Legacy And After-Death

What do you want for your funeral or memorial? (Burial or cremation? Religious or secular? Large or small?)

What do you want others to know or remember about you?

Is there anything you want me to share with specific people after you die?

Are there specific items you'd like to give to certain people?

9. The One Essential Question

If you could ask only ONE question, ask this:

If you were dying and unable to speak for yourself, what would you want me to know?

This question:

- Opens the door.
- Encourages them to share what matters most

- Let's them prioritize
- Provides them with control

Everything else flows from this.

How To Ask The Questions

Pacing

Don't ask all questions in one sitting.

Break into multiple conversations:

- Conversation 1: General philosophy (quality of life, treatment philosophy)
- Conversation 2: Specific scenarios (CPR, ventilator, location)
- Conversation 3: Spirituality and legacy

Or address questions as they become relevant to current health.

Tone

Ask with:

- Curiosity (not judgment)
- Calmness (not anxiety)
- Openness (not agenda)

Your tone says: "I want to understand YOU, not convince you of anything."

Follow-Up

After they answer, dig deeper:

Help me understand why that's important to you. Can you give an example of what that looks like? What if [related scenario], would your answer change?

Deep understanding requires follow-up.

Documentation

As you ask: Take notes during or right after.

Write down:

- Question asked
- Their answer
- Any qualifications or conditions
- Date of conversation

Immediately after:

- Write up notes while fresh
- Share with them: "Is this accurate?"
- Update legal documents to match

The Conversation Map

A proposed outline for an in-depth conversation (90-120 minutes):

Opening (5 min): "I want to understand what's important to you."

Values (15 min): What makes life worth living? Priority ranking?

Treatment Philosophy (15 min): Aggressive or comfort care? CPR? Ventilator? Feeding tube?

Location/Presence (10 min): Where? Who's with you?

Fears (10 min): What are you afraid of? How can I prevent it?

Spiritual (10 min): Religious beliefs affecting care? Rituals?

Practical (10 min): Healthcare proxy? DNR? Organ donation?

Legacy (10 min): What do you want people to know? Messages for specific people?

Closing (5 min): "Thank you. I'll document everything. We can update anytime."

It can be broken into multiple conversations.

Quick Reference: Most Critical Questions

If time is limited, prioritize these six:

1. Would you choose aggressive treatment or comfort care if you had a terminal illness?
2. If your heart stopped, would you want CPR?
3. Where do you want to be? Who do you want with you?
4. Who do you want making decisions if you can't?
5. What are you most afraid of about dying?
6. If you were dying and unable to speak, what would you want me to know?

These six cover the essentials.

"The questions you don't ask today become the decisions you can't make tomorrow".

CHAPTER 8:

Documenting Everything:
Making Wishes Legal and Accessible

―――――――――― ◆◗●◗◆ ――――――――――

The File That Saved Everything

When James had a severe stroke at home, his wife Karen hurried to the hospital. The ER doctor approached her: "Your husband can't breathe on his own. We need to intubate. Should we proceed?" Karen reached into her purse and pulled out a laminated card. "Here's his advance directive. He explicitly stated no intubation if he's in a vegetative state. The neurologist confirmed extensive brain damage with little chance of recovery. So, no—respect his wishes." The doctor examined the card, signed, witnessed, and dated six months earlier. "I understand. We'll keep him comfortable." James died peacefully six hours later. Karen stayed with him, confident she'd honored his wishes precisely because he had documented them.

Why Documentation Matters

Conversations are essential. But they aren't sufficient.

Why:

- Memory fades (after 6 months, you remember 30% of details)
- Family disputes cannot be verified without documentation.
- Medical staff requires proof; verbal wishes are not sufficient for legal decisions.
- State laws differ (some mandate particular legal forms)
- Crises happen quickly (no time to call family and discuss).

Documentation turns wishes into enforceable decisions.

The Essential Documents

1. Living Will (Advance Directive)

What it is: A legal document that states which treatments you want or do not want if you are terminally ill or permanently unconscious.

What it covers: CPR, ventilator, feeding tube, dialysis, antibiotics, pain management, organ donation.

When it activates: Only when you cannot speak and meet specific conditions (terminal, permanent unconsciousness, end-stage).

Who needs one: Everyone 18+

2. Healthcare Power Of Attorney (Healthcare Proxy)

What it is: Identifies a specific person authorized to make medical decisions for you if you are unable to do so.

What they can do:

- Consent to or refuse treatment
- Select doctors and facilities
- Access medical records.
- Enforce your living will.

Who to choose: Someone you trust, who knows your wishes, can handle stress, and will advocate even when difficult.

Name backups: Primary plus two alternates

When it activates: When your doctor certifies you can't make decisions (unconscious, confused, incapacitated).

Who needs one: Everyone 18+

THIS IS THE MOST IMPORTANT DOCUMENT.

3. DNR (Do Not Resuscitate)

What it is: Medical order indicating no CPR if the heart or breathing stops.

Two types:

- Hospital DNR: Valid only within that facility.
- Out-of-hospital DNR (POLST): Recognized everywhere, portable

What DNR does NOT mean: It does NOT mean "do not treat"; you still receive all other care.

What DNR DOES mean: No chest compressions, no electric shocks, no breathing tube. Natural death occurs.

How to obtain one: Request it from your doctor.

Who needs one: Anyone with a terminal illness or anyone who doesn't want CPR.

4. Polst (Physician Orders For Life-Sustaining Treatment)

What it is: More detailed medical orders than DNR

What it covers: CPR (yes/no), medical interventions (comfort/limited/full), antibiotics, IV fluids, feeding tube, hospitalization.

Key difference:

- Living Will = your preferences
- POLST = doctor's orders based on your preferences (immediately actionable)

How to obtain one: Talk with your doctor and complete it together.

Who needs one: Anyone with a serious illness or an elderly person seeking treatment limits.

5. Organ Donation

How to document:

- Driver's license (check donor box)
- State Registry (Online)
- Include in an advance directive.

Options: All organs, specific organs, transplant only, research only, don't donate

Important: Family members can usually override, so communicate your wishes clearly to them.

How To Create These Documents

Living Will & Healthcare Power of Attorney

Step 1: Get the form

Options:

- Download state-specific form (Google "[your state] living will")
- Use national form: CaringInfo.org
- Work with attorney ($100-300)
- Online service like LegalZoom ($20-100)

Step 2: Complete the form

Be specific:

✓ **Good:** "If I am in a persistent vegetative state with no hope of recovery, I do NOT want: CPR, ventilator, feeding tube. I want comfort care only."

✗ **Too vague:** "I want reasonable medical treatment."

Step 3: Sign and witness

Usually requires:

- Your signature
- Two witnesses (not your proxy or family members)
- Notary (required in some states, not in others)

Check your state's specific requirements.

Step 4: Distribute copies (see below)

DNR / POLST

You cannot make these yourself. Your doctor has to write them.

Process:

1. Talk to the doctor: "I don't want CPR if my heart stops. Can you write a DNR?"
2. The doctor fills out and signs the official form.
3. Obtain multiple copies.
4. Keep the original with you at all times (if you're at home)
5. Out-of-hospital DNR: Bright-colored wallet card or bracelet, visible to EMTs

Where To Store Documents

The most effective advance directive is useless if no one can locate it.

Physical copies:

- Originals: Fireproof safe at home (NOT a safe deposit box, can't be accessed quickly))
- Tell the family the exact location.

- Wallet card: "I have an advance directive. Contact [proxy] at [phone]."

Digital copies:

- Secure cloud storage options (Google Drive, Dropbox, password-protected)
- Tell the family how to access.

Who Needs Copies

ESSENTIAL (must have):

☐ Healthcare proxy (primary and backups)
☐ Your primary care doctor
☐ Your home (specific location family knows)

RECOMMENDED:

☐ Adult children / close family
☐ The hospital you use frequently
☐ Nursing home / assisted living (if applicable)
☐ Your attorney

OPTIONAL:

☐ State registry (if available)
☐ Clergy
☐ Close friends

Emergency Access

Create emergency info sheet:

EMERGENCY MEDICAL INFORMATION

[Your Name]

I HAVE AN ADVANCE DIRECTIVE

Healthcare Proxy: [Name, Phone]

Documents Location: [Specific location]

Key Wishes: DNR: YES/NO

Contact [proxy] BEFORE major decisions

Doctor: [Name, Phone]

Post on the refrigerator. EMTs check there.
Keep a copy in your wallet.

Keeping Documents Updated

Advance directives need updating.

When to Update

- Diagnosis of a serious illness
- Significant health change
- Marriage, divorce, and remarriage
- Death of Healthcare Proxy
- Relocate to a different state
- Change of wishes

Also: Review every 2-5 years minimum (annually recommended)

How to Update

Create new document:

1. Fill out the new form.
2. Sign and witness.
3. Distribute new copies.
4. Mark new document: "This supersedes all previous directives dated [old date]."
5. Destroy or label old copies as "VOID."

Special Considerations

If You Have Dementia

Do this NOW while you have capacity:

- Complete all documents
- Video yourself explaining wishes (proves capacity)
- Have the doctor assess and document capacity
- Be extra specific

After capacity lost: Too late. Whatever you had before stands.

If You're Traveling

Carry:

- Wallet card containing emergency information
- Copy of advance directive
- Contact information for proxy

Consider:

- Medical alert bracelet (if DNR)
- Translation if international

If You Move States

Important: Directives are state-specific.

If you move:

- Obtain new forms for the new state.
- Complete and distribute.
- Don't assume the old directive remains valid.

HIPAA Authorization

Include in Healthcare POA:

I authorize my healthcare proxy to access all of my medical records, including those protected by HIPAA.

Without this, doctors might withhold information even from your proxy.

The Documentation Checklist

Documents Created:

- ☐ Living Will (completed, signed, witnessed)
- ☐ Healthcare Power of Attorney (completed, signed, witnessed)
- ☐ DNR order (if applicable)
- ☐ POLST form (if applicable)
- ☐ Organ donation (registered)

Documents Stored:

- ☐ Originals stored in a fireproof safe at home
- ☐ Location known to family
- ☐ Digital copies stored in a secure cloud

Documents Distributed:

- ☐ Healthcare proxy has a copy
- ☐ Alternate proxies have copies
- ☐ Primary doctor has a copy
- ☐ Adult children and family have copies
- ☐ Facility has a copy (if applicable)

State Requirements Met:

☐ Verified state-specific requirements
☐ Appropriate witnesses used
☐ Notarized when necessary

Emergency Access:

☐ Wallet card created.
☐ Emergency info sheet on refrigerator.
☐ Family knows the location of the documents.

Review Schedule:

☐ Annual review date scheduled
☐ Calendar reminder set

Communication:

☐ Healthcare proxy understands your wishes in detail
☐ Family has discussed your wishes
☐ Doctor has discussed your wishes

The Bottom Line

Conversations express wishes.

Documentation makes those wishes enforceable. Both are crucial. Make the documents. Store them properly. Distribute copies. Keep them up to date. This is non-negotiable. Your wishes on paper hold more power than your family's memory of them.

"Document your wishes. Your family will thank you when it matters most".

PART THREE:

UNDERSTANDING YOUR OPTIONS

CHAPTER 9:

Understanding Hospice:
What It Is and Who Provides It

―――――――――◆●◆―――――――――

The Myth That Kills

When Dr. Anderson suggested hospice for Margaret's father's end-stage heart failure, Margaret responded immediately: "Absolutely not. We're not giving up. We're going to fight this."

So, they pursued treatments. For three months, her father endured four hospitalizations, constant pain, severe nausea, and complete exhaustion. He spent his final months undergoing treatments that brought weeks of misery rather than months of life.

Finally, as he was actively dying, the doctor said, "It's time for hospice."

Hospice was arranged. Within 24 hours, pain was managed, breathing became easier, and he was alert enough to talk with his family. He smiled for the first time in weeks.

"Why didn't we do this sooner?" Margaret asked.

"Because you thought hospice meant giving up," the nurse said. "It doesn't. It means shifting from cure to comfort. Your father could have had three peaceful months instead of three months of suffering."

This is the cost of not understanding hospice.

What Hospice Actually Means

In twenty years of hospice nursing, I've seen the same pattern happen hundreds of times: families wait too long because they misunderstand what hospice really provides. They believe they're "giving up" by calling hospice, so they delay. They wait and wait until the patient becomes so sick, so exhausted, and so overwhelmed by symptoms that there's barely any time left to enjoy. Then, when hospice finally begins, I hear nearly the same comment every time: "I wish we'd done this sooner." Let me clear up the myths that cause families to delay.

Myth #1: "Hospice Is Giving Up"

This is the biggest misconception, and it harms people. Hospice isn't giving up; it's shifting goals from cure to comfort. You're not doing nothing; you're doing different things: active medical care focused on making you comfortable, expert symptom management, twenty-four-hour support, and a whole team working together. Think of it like this: you're running a marathon, and you realize you can't win. You have two choices: keep sprinting until you collapse, miserable and exhausted, or adjust your pace, enjoy the scenery, and finish strong. That's not giving up; that's wisdom.

Myth #2: "Hospice Means You Have Days Left"

People often think hospice is only for the final 48 hours, but that's not true. Hospice is for anyone with a prognosis of six months or less; six months, not six days. The reality is that the median hospice stay in America is just 18 days, which is shockingly short. Why? Because families tend to wait until the very last minute, assuming hospice is only for imminent death. However, many people don't realize that about 15% of hospice patients live longer than six months, and that's perfectly okay. If you improve, you can "graduate" from hospice; it's not a one-way door. Experts like me, who work in this every day, recommend starting hospice when the prognosis is six months, not six days, because that's when you truly benefit from everything hospice has to offer.

Myth #3: "Hospice Hastens Death"

I hear this fear all the time: "If we stop treatment, won't she die faster?" Actually, no. Research shows hospice patients often live as long or longer than similar patients who receive aggressive treatment. Why? Because when you're not fighting treatments, not rushing to appointments, and not enduring side effects, your body can often rally. Less stress. Better symptom management. Better nutrition. Better sleep. Emotional peace. All of this makes a difference. Hospice allows for natural death when the body is ready. We don't give medications to hasten death. We don't withdraw food or water. We don't withhold the treatment you want. We simply stop treatments that cause suffering without providing benefit.

Myth #4: "Hospice Is A Place"

When people hear "hospice," they picture a building. But hospice is a service, not a location. Sixty-five percent of hospice care occurs at home. In your own bed. In your own space. The team comes to you. Twenty percent happens in nursing homes or assisted living, wherever you already live. Ten percent takes place in dedicated hospice facilities. Five percent occurs in hospitals. Most of the time, you don't go anywhere. We come to you.

Myth #5: "Hospice Is Only For Cancer"

Cancer is common in hospice, but it's not the only qualifying diagnosis. Any terminal illness qualifies: heart failure, COPD, dementia, kidney or liver failure, ALS, stroke; anything with a prognosis of six months or less. If your body is shutting down and a cure isn't possible, hospice is an option.

Myth #6: "Hospice Is Expensive"

This one surprises people: Hospice is almost entirely covered by insurance. Medicare, which covers most hospice patients, pays for everything— all services, all medications related to your diagnosis, all equipment, and all supplies. It also includes twenty-four-hour support, respite care so your family can rest, and even bereavement counseling for your family after you die. Typical family cost: zero to fifty dollars a month, mostly for medication copays. Compare that to an ICU stay costing ten to thirty thousand dollars per day or chemotherapy at the same monthly range. Hospice is not only better for quality of life; it's also more affordable.

Myth #7: "You Can't Have Any Treatment"

People often think hospice means no treatment at all. That's not true. You can receive any treatment aimed at comfort, such as pain medications, breathing treatments, oxygen, antibiotics if they improve comfort, blood transfusions if they make you feel better, radiation for pain relief, physical therapy to help you move more comfortably, and wound care. What you can't have are treatments intended to cure that cause suffering, like curative chemotherapy, curative radiation, curative surgery, ICU care for a terminal condition, or usually dialysis. The key question is always: Is this for comfort or cure? If it's for comfort, hospice covers it.

Myth #8: "You'll Be Drugged And Unconscious"

Families worry: "They're going to dope her up until she's gone." That's not the goal. The goal is to provide comfort AND awareness. We want you to be pain-free or nearly pain-free, around two or three out of ten on the pain scale. You should be alert enough to interact with family and comfortable enough to enjoy your time. Most hospice patients are not heavily sedated. Some require deep sedation if symptoms become unbearable, but this is uncommon and always discussed with family beforehand. We adjust medications based on your preferences. Want to be more alert despite some pain? We can do that. Need less pain but more drowsiness? We can do that too. You stay in control.

When Hospice Works Beautifully

Let me tell you about Emma.

She was seventy-eight with end-stage COPD. Her pulmonologist said, "You have maybe six months. We can keep trying treatments, or you can choose hospice." Emma chose hospice immediately. "I'm tired of hospitals," she said. "I want to be home." We started hospice on a Tuesday. By Thursday, her breathing was better managed with oxygen and medications adjusted just for her. By the following week, she had energy she hadn't felt in months. No more emergency room visits. No more panic about whether she could catch her breath. For the next four months, Emma lived fully. She hosted Sunday dinners, small ones, but she was there. She taught her granddaughter to knit. She sat in her garden every morning with coffee, something she'd been too short of breath to do for years.

When I visited for our regular check-ins, she'd smile and say, "Best decision I ever made. I thought hospice meant dying. Turns out it meant living."

She died peacefully in her sleep on a Sunday morning, in her own bed, five months after starting hospice. Her family told me later: "Those five months were a gift. She was really there in a way she hadn't been for years. Just Mom, comfortable, present, herself." That's what hospice done right looks like.

How Hospice Actually Works

Hospice began with a simple idea from Dame Cicely Saunders, a British nurse: "You matter to the end of your life. We'll help you die peacefully and live until you die." In 1982, Medicare introduced a hospice benefit. To qualify, you need three things: a terminal illness with a prognosis of six months or less, certification by two physicians, your doctor and a hospice physician, and a choice of comfort over cure. Once you qualify, you receive four levels of care based on your needs.

Routine home care is the most common. The hospice team visits you wherever you live. Most days, you're on your own with family, but the team is available by phone anytime and visits regularly.

Continuous home care occurs during a crisis, with a nurse staying in your home for eight to twenty-four hours to manage severe symptoms. After the crisis passes, you resume routine care.

Inpatient respite gives your exhausted family a break. You stay at a facility for up to five days while your family rests, then you return home.

General inpatient is for severe symptom crises that can't be managed at home. You go to a hospice facility or hospital until symptoms are controlled, then usually return home.

Most people remain on routine home care throughout.

Who Takes Care Of You

You don't just get one person; you get a whole team. When hospice care started for Mr. Chen, his wife expected just one nurse to visit occasionally. Instead, she had nine people working together. Let me walk you through who showed up and what they did.

First was Sarah, the registered nurse. She served as their case manager, the main contact who coordinated everything. During her initial visit, she spent three hours conducting a thorough assessment, reviewing his medications, ordering equipment like a hospital bed and oxygen, and teaching Mrs. Chen what to expect and how to care for him. After that, Sarah visited two to three times a week, more when necessary, and she was available by phone around the clock.

Dr. Williams, the hospice physician, oversaw all medical care. He only visited twice during the entire hospice stay, but reviewed Mr. Chen's case weekly, approved medication changes, and was available if Sarah needed medical backup.

A hospice aide came three times a week to help with bathing and personal care. This wasn't medical treatment; it was dignity care, to keep Mr. Chen feeling clean and comfortable and ease some of the burden on his wife.

The social worker, Rachel, visited to assist with practical issues like insurance questions, advance directive paperwork, family conflicts, and connecting with community resources.

The chaplain stopped by not to convert anyone but to offer spiritual support if needed. When Mrs. Chen mentioned she was Catholic but hadn't attended church in years, the chaplain arranged for her priest to visit and give Mr. Chen the last rites. It brought her great peace.

A volunteer came once a week to sit with Mr. Chen while Mrs. Chen went grocery shopping or out to lunch with a friend. These volunteers weren't medical professionals; they were trained community members offering companionship and support.

When Mr. Chen's pain became harder to control, a specialized pain management consultant temporarily joined the team to adjust medications until they found the right combination.

The dietitian helped when Mr. Chen's appetite decreased by suggesting minor adjustments, such as smoothies instead of full meals and favorite foods rather than "healthy" options.

The bereavement counselor supported Mrs. Chen for thirteen months after Mr. Chen passed away. Phone calls, support groups, and individual counseling helped her navigate grief.

All of this, including every person, visit, and service, was covered by Medicare. Mrs. Chen paid nothing. That's how hospice care operates. It's not just one nurse visiting occasionally, but a whole team supporting you.

What Hospice Provides

When Sarah delivered supplies to the Chen house, Mrs. Chen was surprised. "All of this is included?" A hospital bed so Mr. Chen could be positioned comfortably. An oxygen concentrator and portable tank. A walker. A wheelchair for later. A bedside commode. Incontinence supplies. Wound care supplies. Everything they'd need.

The medications followed, all connected to his diagnosis: pain meds, nausea meds, anxiety meds, and breathing treatments. No copays.

But what surprised Mrs. Chen the most was the 24-hour nurse line. When Mr. Chen's breathing suddenly worsened at three in the morning, she called. A nurse guided her through it, assessed her over the phone, and sent a nurse to her house within an hour.

I thought we'd be alone, she told me later. "We weren't. Ever." That's what hospice offers. Not just equipment and medications, but peace of mind.

The Biggest Mistake Families Make

The biggest mistake isn't choosing hospice; it's waiting too long to decide. The pattern I most often see: family waits until the patient has only days left, then finally agrees to hospice, and we rush to get everything in place. The patient dies forty-eight hours later. And the family says, "I wish we'd done this sooner." Every single time.

Because here's what happens when you procrastinate: You end up managing crises. We address symptoms in the final days and support the family through active dying. That's valuable.

But here's what you're really missing: time. Not necessarily longer life, but more meaningful time. Time when the patient feels comfortable enough to be present, alert enough to speak, and strong enough to say what needs to be said.

Families who contact hospice early, when the prognosis is months instead of days, gain something priceless. They cherish afternoons in the garden, birthday parties, reconciliation talks, last fishing trips, and the memories made while the patient is still healthy enough to participate. The families who wait get none of that.

So, when is the right time for hospice? It's when the prognosis is six months or less and a cure isn't possible. Not when you're down to forty-eight hours. It's when you still have time to live, not just time to die.

Common Questions

Can we try treatment first and do hospice later? You can. But remember: if you spend three months on treatment that doesn't work, you've lost three months of comfort. If treatment genuinely helps and gives you meaningful additional time, then it was worthwhile. But if it doesn't, you've traded comfort for suffering with no benefits. The question is: What are the chances that treatment will actually help versus cause harm?

What if we choose hospice and then change our minds? You can leave hospice anytime. If you improve, want to try treatment again, or just aren't ready, you can revoke. About seven percent of patients do. Some come back to hospice later. Some don't. It's your choice.

Can hospice do anything in a nursing home?
Yes. Hospice services are available wherever you are, whether in a nursing home, assisted living, or your own home. The hospice team works with facility staff to coordinate care.

How do we find a good hospice? Ask your doctor for recommendations. Find out which hospices local hospitals routinely work with. Request a list of area hospices from Medicare and review their quality ratings online. Interview two or three before making a decision. Inquire about the number of patients they serve, their nurse-to-patient ratios, and their response time to after-hours calls. Not all hospices are equal. Do your research.

"Hospice doesn't mean giving up on life. It means death is approaching, and you choose comfort instead of suffering. That's not a weakness. That's wisdom".

CHAPTER 10:

Quality vs. Quantity:
The Fundamental Trade-Off

The Two Paths

Tom had stage 4 pancreatic cancer. His oncologist, Dr. Patel, laid out two options at their last appointment.

"We can try aggressive chemotherapy," she said. "Success rate is about fifteen percent. If it works, you might get three to six extra months. But the side effects will be severe: nausea, fatigue, and constant hospital visits. Your quality of life will be minimal."

Tom listened. Or, "Dr. Patel continued, "you can choose hospice, comfort care. You'll probably have two to four months, but you'll be comfortable. At home. With energy to enjoy your family."

Tom didn't hesitate. "I've been fighting for two years. I'm tired. I'll take three good months over six bad ones."

He spent those three months at home. His granddaughter was born during that time. He held her every single day, sitting in his favorite chair by the window. His last words, whispered to his daughter: "I made the right choice."

This chapter is about making the right decision for yourself.

The Fundamental Trade-Off

Here's what I need you to understand: At the end of life, you cannot maximize both quality and quantity. You have to choose. You can focus on quantity, pursue every treatment, accept every side effect, and hope for more time. Or you can focus on quality, seek comfort, minimize suffering, and get the most value from your remaining time. Neither choice is wrong, but they are very different. Most people don't realize they're making this decision. They believe aggressive treatment will give them both more time and better-quality time, but it rarely does. Aggressive treatment at the end of life often only prolongs the dying process, not the living. It causes suffering without offering significant benefit. Usually, it happens in hospitals, not homes. And it can leave you too sick to enjoy whatever extra time you might gain.

The question you need to ask isn't "Will treatment give me more time?" The real question is: "Will treatment give me more good time, or just more time?" That's a very different question.

Wrong Reasons And Right Reasons

I've sat with hundreds of patients facing this exact choice. And what I've learned is this: There's no single right answer. But there are wrong reasons for choosing. Wrong reason to choose treatment: "My family will think I gave up."

Right reason to choose treatment: "I genuinely want to try. I'll regret it if I don't." Wrong reason to choose hospice: "Everyone says I should stop fighting."

Right reason to choose hospice: "I'm exhausted. I want peace." The difference is: Whose choice is it? The saddest deaths I've seen weren't the ones where treatment failed. They were the ones where patients never made their own choice. They chose treatment to please their children. Or they decided on hospice because their doctor seemed to want them to. Either way, they died with someone else's decision, not their own.

Here's the core question: If you knew for sure that you'd die in three months, no matter what, would you still opt for treatment?

If the answer is no, you're choosing treatment for the wrong reasons.

If the answer is yes, because trying matters to you, because exhausting options brings you peace, because you need to know you did everything, then choose treatment with my blessing. Just make sure it's your choice.

Two Patients, Two Choices, Both Right

Let me tell you about Janet and Robert. I cared for both of them during the same month, and their stories showed me that opposite choices can both be right.

Janet was sixty-four and fighting stage 4 lung cancer. Her oncologist said, "Chemotherapy might give you three to four more months. The success rate is about twenty percent. Side effects will be significant."

Janet said right away, "I'm doing it. My son is getting married in five months. I have to be there."

She went through six weeks of harsh chemotherapy, losing all her hair and feeling nauseous constantly. She was hospitalized twice for dehydration. Her family wanted her to stop; they hated seeing her suffer.

But Janet refused to quit. "Just get me to the wedding," she said. The tumor shrank. She made it. Walked her son down the aisle, bald under a beautiful scarf, so weak she could barely stand but radiant with purpose. She died two weeks later.

At her funeral, her son said through tears, "She fought for me. She suffered for me. That's love." Janet prioritized quantity; she needed those extra weeks to attend that wedding. The suffering was worth it to her because she got what she needed: to see her son married.

Robert was sixty-six with stage 4 colon cancer. His oncologist gave him the same speech: "Chemo might give you three to four more months. The success rate is about twenty percent. Side effects will be significant." Robert said, "No. I've been fighting for two years. I'm done. I want to go home." His children panicked. "Dad, you have to try! You can't give up!" Robert was firm. "I'm not giving up. I'm choosing something better."

He went on hospice, and something surprising happened. Within two weeks, his energy returned. He wasn't cured; the cancer was still there, but he wasn't being poisoned by chemotherapy either. He spent three months fishing, something he hadn't been able to do during treatment because he was too sick. He taught his ten-year-old grandson everything he knew about casting, patience, and reading the water. One morning, they caught a twelve-pound bass. Robert had that fish mounted, and his grandson still has it. Every morning, Robert sat on his dock with coffee, watching the sun come up. "I haven't felt this good in two years," he told me during one of my visits. He died peacefully at home, exactly three months after stopping treatment.

At his funeral, his grandson, now a teenager, said: "Grandpa taught me to fish in his last months. Every time I go to the lake, I remember him. That's love." Robert chose quality; he traded potential extra time for guaranteed comfortable time. For him, three months fishing beat six months being sick. Both chose love. Janet's love looked like fighting to be present. Robert's love looked like it was stopping the fight from being present differently. Neither was wrong.

How To Think About Your Choice

Let me walk you through the questions that help clarify what's right for you. Not what's right in general, but what's right for you specifically.

Start with what makes your life worth living.

Not the big, abstract things. The small daily moments. Morning coffee on the porch. Reading to your grandchildren, working in the garden, Sunday dinners with family, watching birds at the feeder; consider what truly matters. Now ask yourself: Will treatment let me continue these things, or will it stop me? If chemotherapy causes you to be too nauseated to enjoy coffee, too fatigued to read, or too sick to have Sunday dinner, you've traded what makes life meaningful for more time being technically alive but not truly living. That might be worth it if treatment offers a real chance at a cure or a meaningful extension of life. But if you're exchanging three good months for six miserable months, that math doesn't add up for most people.

Next, figure out what you're willing to trade for more time.

Be clear about your limits.

Some people tell me, "I'll trade nausea and fatigue. But not my mind. If chemo causes confusion, I stop." Others say: "I'll trade everything, nausea, pain, hospitalization, all of it, for any chance at my daughter's wedding in six months."

There's no one-size-fits-all answer, but you should know your limits before you're in a crisis, especially since doctors are asking you to make quick decisions.

Then sit with the central question: Quality or quantity, if you can only choose one?

Most people answer this too quickly. Sit with it for days, not minutes. Imagine both scenarios vividly: six more months, mostly in hospitals, nauseated, exhausted, but alive; or three more months, mostly at home, comfortable, present, but shorter. Which scenario, when you really imagine it, makes your heart feel more at peace?

Be honest about who you're doing this for.

This is difficult, but essential. Many people seek treatment not for themselves but to satisfy their family, to prevent disappointing their spouse, or because of cultural pressure to "fight." They believe that "quitters" choose comfort. But this is your life, your death, your body. Your family will grieve either way. It's better they mourn your death than watch you endure treatment you never wanted just to make them think you fought hard enough.

Finally, think about regret.

Which could you regret more? Choosing treatment, enduring suffering, and facing the possibility that it might not work, then wishing you'd picked a more convenient time? Or opting for comfort, dying sooner, and wishing you'd tried treatment? Which regret can you live with or accept? There's no right or wrong answer; just your answer.

Understanding Statistics (What Doctors Mean)

When your doctor says "average survival eight months," here's what that actually means: Some people in the study lived two months. Others lived eighteen months. You won't know which category you're in until you try.

When they say "thirty percent success rate," they mean thirty out of one hundred people respond to treatment. Seventy out of one hundred don't. And "response" might just mean the tumor shrinks, not that you're cured. Even the responders eventually die.

Here's the harsh reality: Side effects are guaranteed. Benefits are not.

One hundred percent of people who undergo chemotherapy experience side effects. Only thirty percent see benefits.

You're guaranteed to suffer. The benefit is a gamble.

That doesn't mean you shouldn't try. It just means you need to go in with your eyes open.

The "Try It And See" Approach

Some people can't choose between treatment and comfort without trying first. That's okay. There's a middle way.

Try treatment for a set period with clear decision points.

Example: "I'll try chemotherapy for two cycles, six weeks. If the tumor shrinks and side effects are tolerable, I'll continue. If the tumor isn't responding or side effects are unbearable, I'll stop and switch to hospice."

This approach gives you a chance to try without committing to suffering indefinitely if it's not working.

The key is to communicate this plan to your family now: "I'm going to try this treatment. But if it's not working or it's too hard, I'm going to stop. I need you to support that decision when the time comes."

Set the expectation early. It makes stopping much easier when needed.

What Doctors Wish You Understood

Most oncologists will continue offering treatment until you explicitly tell them to stop. That's their job, to give you options. But options don't mean they are recommending those options.

If you privately asked your oncologist, off the record, "What would you do in my position?", many would answer, "I'd probably choose hospice." They observe how aggressive treatments affect quality of life and how rarely they provide meaningful benefits at the end stages.

However, they can't state this officially. They must offer you all available options.

You have to be the one to say, "enough."

Here's something else doctors know but rarely say directly: Hospice patients often live as long as, or longer than, those undergoing aggressive treatments. Why? Because of reduced stress, better symptom control, improved nutrition, better sleep, and emotional peace, all of which contribute to this outcome.

The best time for hospice isn't when you're actively dying. The median hospice stay in America is eighteen days, which is too short. Ideally, it should be two to three months, providing enough time to fully benefit from comfort care.

When Quality Makes More Sense

Consider choosing quality and comfort when:

- Success rates are below twenty percent.
- Extra time would be just a few weeks, not months.
- Your current quality of life remains good (you feel alright now and don't want to trade that).
- You have time-sensitive goals (wedding in two months; might not survive treatment to reach them)
- Treatment would involve extensive hospitalization.
- You're exhausted from fighting (been in treatment for over two years).
- Your gut says: "I'd prefer three good months over six bad ones."

When Quantity Makes More Sense

Consider choosing treatment when:

- Success rates range from moderate to high (over forty percent).
- Extra time could be substantial (several months to years)
- You have something special to look forward to, like your daughter's wedding in eight months.
- The side effects are manageable for you.
- You're not prepared to accept death (you need to explore all options first for your own peace).
- New or experimental treatments are accessible.
- Your gut says: "I'll try anything if there's a chance."

Both Choices Can Be Right

I cared for Sarah, fifty-two, who chose experimental treatment with a twenty percent success rate. It worked, and she lived four more years. She saw both her kids graduate from high school. Eventually, the disease progressed, and she died. But those four years mattered.

Her reflection, recorded in hospice: "Brutal. Worth it. No regrets."

I cared for Tom, sixty-eight, who decided to enter hospice immediately. He spent three peaceful months at home, holding his newborn granddaughter every day. He died peacefully in his own bed.

His reflection, shared with me during our final visit: "Best three months of my life. Perfect ending."

Both were right for themselves.

"The right choice is the one that aligns with your values, not your family's fear, not your doctor's default, not society's expectations. Your values. Your choice".

CHAPTER 11:

Where You Want to Die: Understanding Your Options

―――――――――― ◆◗●◖◆ ――――――――――

The Question That Matters

Patricia was eighty-two and suffering from end-stage heart failure. When the hospital doctor told her she needed to stay in the ICU, she looked him directly in the eye and said, "I want to die at home." "You're too sick. You can't leave," he replied. Patricia's voice was calm but resolute. "I'm leaving. Prepare my discharge." The doctor hesitated, citing medical complications and liability, but Patricia remained firm. Six hours later, she was in her own bed with hospice nurses arranging everything. She died peacefully three days afterward, in the bedroom where she had slept for forty years, with her daughter holding one hand and her cat curled beside her other arm. She knew exactly where she wanted to be, and she made it happen.

The Place Doesn't Matter As Much As You Think

I've helped people die in every imaginable setting. Mansions with marble floors. Mobile homes with leaky roofs. Hospice facilities that look like spas. Stark hospital rooms with fluorescent lights. Nursing homes that smell like disinfectant. Tiny apartments where I could barely fit my equipment bag. And here's what I've learned: The place doesn't matter nearly as much as you think. The people do.

I've witnessed peaceful deaths in stark hospital rooms because family was present, love was spoken, and the patient felt surrounded by what mattered. I've seen difficult deaths in beautiful homes because family was fighting, the patient felt like a burden, or symptoms were out of control, and everyone was panicking.

So, when people ask me, "What's the best place to die?" I tell them the truth: The real question isn't "Where do you want to die?" It's "Where can you have the death you want?"

For some people, that's home. In their own bed, with their dog at their feet, looking at their garden through the window, sleeping under the quilt their grandmother made.

For others, it's a hospice facility. Where round-the-clock professional care means family can just be family instead of caregivers. Where they can leave for a few hours without guilt because trained staff is there.

For others, it's wherever they are when death occurs. A nursing home they've lived in for years and call home. A hospital where symptoms finally overwhelm them.
All of these can be good deaths if they align with what matters most to you.

The Four Options

Let me show you what each option actually looks like.

Home

This is what most people say they want. About sixty-five to seventy percent of Americans, when asked, say they want to die at home. Here's how it works: The hospice team comes to you. They deliver all the equipment: hospital bed, oxygen, wheelchair, supplies. Your family provides the day-to-day care with the team's support and guidance. A nurse visits two to three times a week, sometimes more. A hospice aide helps with bathing. The team is available by phone twenty-four hours a day.

What makes home special: it's familiar, comfortable, and free from visitor restrictions; people can come and go as they please. Your pets are there. You have your own food, your own bed, and your own routines. Family intimacy that isn't possible in institutions.

What makes home hard: Families provide caregiving, including not just emotional support but also physical tasks like lifting, toileting, and medication management. This can be exhausting, so you need space and a capable family willing to help. And you need symptoms that can be managed without hospital-level resources. The reality check: Home death requires significant family support. If you live alone, if family is far away or unable to help physically, or if symptoms become complex, staying at home might not be feasible. And that's okay.

Hospital

Some people die in acute care hospitals. They either are already there when death becomes imminent, or symptoms become severe enough to need hospital-level care.

What hospitals provide: Immediate medical support. Expert staff available instantly. No burden on family for physical care; nurses handle everything. All the equipment you might need is right there.

What makes hospitals difficult: Unfamiliarity. Institutional environment. Visiting hours and restrictions. Loss of control, you're told when to eat and sleep. Hospitals are designed for cure, not for comfort or quality of life. Even with a hospice consult, a hospital death can feel clinical rather than peaceful.

The pattern I observe: People end up in hospitals not because they choose to, but because symptoms become uncontrollable at home, leading to a call to 911. Then they are stuck there. If you absolutely want to avoid dying in a hospital, plan ahead. Make sure your family knows: Don't call 911 unless you've agreed to it. Call hospice instead.

Hospice Facility

This is different from a hospital and from a nursing home. It's a dedicated hospice facility, purpose-built for end-of-life care. These facilities are usually small, with eight to twenty beds. They look and feel more like a cozy home than an institution. Every room has space for the family to stay overnight if they want. There's a kitchen where the family can cook, and sometimes there's a garden or patio.

103

Here's what makes them special: 24/7 expert hospice care, a home-like environment, and flexible family visits, whether they want to stay or leave. Family can visit anytime, even at two in the morning, with no restrictions. They can just be family, not caregivers, while someone else manages medications, toileting, and physical care.

The limitation: Not every area has one. They're usually for short-term stays, a few days to a few weeks, when symptoms need intensive management. Ask your hospice if this is available in your area.

I tell families: This is often the best of both worlds. Professional care in a peaceful setting. But it's not available everywhere.

Nursing Home Or Assisted Living

If you're already living in a facility when you go on hospice, you can usually stay there. The hospice team visits the facility and works with the staff there.

What makes this work: It's already familiar. You've been there for months or years. It IS home to you. There's staff available 24/7. Family doesn't need to provide physical care.

What makes this challenging: Coordination between the facility staff and the hospice team can become complicated. Quality of care varies greatly between facilities; some are excellent, others are poor. The truth: If you've lived there for years, if your friends are nearby, and if you've made it your home, staying can offer more comfort than moving to your daughter's guest bedroom.

Don't assume you have to leave just because you're dying. Sometimes staying is the better choice.

Dorothy's Story

I once cared for a woman named Dorothy, who was eighty-one years old and suffering from end-stage COPD. She had lived alone in a small apartment for thirty years. When she entered hospice care, her son insisted, "Mom's coming to my house to die. I won't let her die alone."

But Dorothy pulled me aside during one of my visits. "I don't want to go to his house. I've lived here thirty years. My cat is here. My things. My independence. I want to die here."

"Have you told him?"

"He'll be hurt."

I helped her have that conversation. She sat her son down and said, "Honey, I love you. But this is my home. I want to die here, with my cat, in my own bed. Please respect that."

Her son was hurt at first. Then he understood. "Okay, Mom. We'll make it work."

For the last three weeks of Dorothy's life, her son visited every single day. Sometimes he stayed overnight on her lumpy couch. The hospice team visited regularly. Dorothy's cat, a grumpy old tabby named Frank, slept on her bed every night. She died peacefully at three in the morning, in her own bed, with Frank purring beside her and her son holding her hand.

At the funeral, her son said: "She taught me that loving someone means honoring their choices, not imposing mine." The right place is the place that respects the patient's wishes, even if it's not what the family would choose.

What To Consider

When thinking about where you want to die, here are the factors that actually matter:

Can your family handle it? Not just emotionally but physically. Can they lift you? Transfer you from bed to chair? Manage medications? Do they have time? Are there enough people to share the burden?

If the answer is no, that doesn't mean they don't love you. It means a facility might be the more realistic choice.

What are your symptoms like? Stable pain that's well-controlled? Minimal nausea? Home works fine. But complex symptoms, severe pain that's hard to manage, frequent vomiting, and bleeding might need facility-level care.

The good news: Symptoms can change, and you can transfer. You're not locked into your initial choice.

Is your home suitable? Do you have space for a hospital bed? Can family easily reach you, or are stairs a barrier? Is it climate-controlled? Is it clean enough for wound care? Sometimes the honest answer is: My home isn't set up for this. And that's okay.

What do you value most? This is the most important question. If you say, "I want to be home," then everyone should work hard to make that happen. If you say, "I don't want to burden my family," then a facility might actually be your true preference, and that's valid too.

You Can Change Your Mind

Nothing is permanent. I often see families shifting between different settings.

Start at home. Symptoms get complex. Transfer to the facility for a few days to control symptoms. Then go back home when things are stable.

Or start at home. The family becomes exhausted. They move to the facility permanently, and everyone feels relieved because it was the right decision.

Or start in a facility. Symptoms get better with good hospice care. Move home because you are now able to.

You're not locked in. This isn't a one-time decision. It's an ongoing choice, influenced by changing circumstances.

Why Most People Don't Get Their Choice

Seventy percent of Americans say they want to die at home, but sixty percent actually die in institutions. Why is there such a gap?

Symptoms become unmanageable at home. The family can't handle the physical or emotional burden. There isn't adequate support. Or, most commonly, there was no planning, so when a crisis hit, 911 was called, and the person ended up dying in a hospital by default, not by choice.

With proper hospice support and advanced planning, more people can die at home. However, facilities and hospitals are also suitable options depending on the situation. There's no wrong answer. Just your answer.

What Makes A Good Death In Any Setting

The best place to die is the one that:

Aligns with your values. If you want to be at home, we work to make that happen. If you prefer professional care, we help find the right facility.

Is medically suitable for your symptoms. Some symptoms require facility-level care; others do not.

Is it practical for your family? Not what they wish they could do, but what they can realistically do without harming themselves.

Provides the support you need, whether that's 24/7 professional care, family closeness, or both.

Enables you to die with comfort and dignity.

A good death can happen anywhere. I have seen it in nearly every setting. The key is: choose intentionally, plan ahead, stay flexible, and clearly communicate what matters most to you.

"The best place to die is wherever you feel safe, comfortable, and loved".

CHAPTER 12:

Your Rights and Choices:
What You Can Control

You Have More Power Than You Think

Remember Patricia from Chapter 11? When the doctor told her she had to stay in the ICU, she said, "I want to go home and die there." "If you leave, you'll die." "I know. That's my choice." The doctor didn't think she had that right. But she did. Her daughter intervened: "Doctor, my mother has decision-making capacity. She understands the consequences. She's choosing to leave. Prepare her discharge." And they had to because Patricia had the law on her side.

The Fundamental Principle

You have the right to make your own medical decisions. Full stop.

This includes:

- Accepting or refusing any treatment
- Choosing between treatment options
- Leaving the hospital against medical advice
- Choosing hospice instead of curative care
- Stopping treatment at any point
- Dying on your own terms

Nobody can force treatment on you if you have capacity. Not your doctor. Not your family. Nobody.

What I Wish Every Patient Knew

I've seen too many patients accept treatment they didn't want because they didn't know they could refuse. They believed the doctor knew best, so I had to follow his advice. Or their family wanted them to fight, so they felt they had no choice. Or if they refused treatment, they'd be abandoned. All of these are false.

Here's the truth: Your body. Your decision. Period. The doctor can recommend. Your family can plead. Insurance may or may not cover it. But if you have capacity, if you can understand the information, see how it applies to you, reason through the decision, and communicate your choice, you get to decide. I've seen patients endure months of harsh chemotherapy because they believed they had to. I've watched patients stay in ICUs on ventilators because they thought they couldn't. leave. I've seen patients suffer because nobody told them the most powerful thing a dying person can say:

"No. I'm done. I want comfort."

And when they finally speak up, when they finally claim their right to refuse, I often see something powerful. Not resignation. Relief. Because dying on your own terms, with your choices respected, is completely different from dying according to someone else's plan.

What "Capacity" Means

Capacity means you can understand information about your condition and options, appreciate how it applies to you personally, reason through the decision, and communicate your choice.

You have capacity even if:

- You're very sick.
- You're in pain.
- You're elderly.
- You make decisions that others believe are "wrong."
- You decide to refuse life-saving treatment.

You lack capacity only if:

- You're unconscious.
- You're severely demented.
- You're delirious or acutely confused.
- You're too confused to reason through information.

If you have capacity, your choice prevails. Always.

Your Rights In Plain Language

You have the right to informed consent. Before any treatment, the medical team must tell you what it is, why they recommend it, what the risks and benefits are, what alternatives exist, and what happens if you refuse. Then you decide.

You have the right to refuse any treatment, including CPR, ventilator, feeding tube, dialysis, chemotherapy, surgery, antibiotics, or hospitalization. Anything. Even if refusing means you might die. Your decision must be respected.

You have the right to leave the hospital. Any time, even "Against Medical Advice." The hospital cannot physically stop you. They'll ask you to sign a form; you can refuse that, too. You're free to leave.

You have the right to choose hospice. When you're eligible for hospice (with a prognosis of six months or less), you can choose it even if your doctor or family objects. You can also revoke hospice at any time, return to treatment, or come back to hospice later. It's your choice.

You have the right to adequate pain management. You don't have to tolerate severe pain just because someone's worried about addiction. At the end of life, addiction isn't relevant. Comfort is what matters.

You have the right to choose who can visit you. You control your visitors, regardless of legal relationships. This is especially important for LGBTQ+ patients, chosen family, and estranged relatives.

You have the right to privacy. The medical team cannot share your information without your permission. You control who has access to details about your condition.

When Doctors Push Back

Sometimes, doctors resist when you refuse treatment or opt for hospice. It happens. Here's what to say:

The doctor says: "You can't refuse this treatment, you'll die."

You say: "I understand the consequences. I have capacity. I'm refusing treatment. Please document my refusal in the chart."

The doctor says: "Let's try one more round of chemotherapy."

You say: "I appreciate your effort, but I'm choosing to stop treatment and start hospice. Please make the hospice referral."

Doctor says: "Your family wants you to keep fighting."

You say: "I have capacity. This is my decision, not theirs. Please honor my choice."

Doctor says: "I think you're giving up too soon."

You say: "I respect your opinion, but this is my body and my life. I'm choosing comfort over cure. If you can't support that decision, I need a different doctor."

The key: Be firm. Don't apologize. Don't over-explain. Clearly state your choice and expect it to be respected.

Common Scenarios And What To Say

Hospital says you can't leave:

"I'm leaving against medical advice. Prepare my discharge paperwork, or I'll walk out without it."

The hospital won't let your partner visit because you're not married.

Federal law requires you to allow visitors I designate, regardless of relationship. If you refuse, I'll file a formal complaint.

Family wants treatment, but you want hospice:

To the doctor: "I have decision-making capacity. I'm choosing hospice. My family's disagreement doesn't change my legal right to make this choice. Please proceed with the hospice referral."

Doctor won't increase pain medication.

My pain is an eight out of ten. I need better control. If you won't provide adequate pain management, I need a referral to a pain specialist.

Nursing facility says they don't allow hospice:

Federal law requires facilities to provide hospice services to residents who qualify. If you refuse, you're violating federal law, and I will report you to Medicare.

When Family Disagrees With Your Choice

This is the scenario that causes the most conflict: You want hospice. Your family wants you to keep fighting. If you have capacity, your choice prevails. Not theirs. Yours.

Here's what to do: Clearly state to your medical team: "I'm choosing hospice. I have decision-making capacity. Please proceed with my choice regardless of my family's objections." Ask the doctor to document this in your chart. If family interferes or tries to override you, you can restrict their access to your medical information. You can even ban them from your hospital room if necessary. Your family's feelings matter. Their fear and grief are real. But your right to decide about your own body matters more.

How To Advocate For Yourself

Be clear and direct. Don't hint or soften your language. Clearly state what you want. Repeat yourself if necessary; if you're ignored the first time, say it again, and again. Put it in writing, as written requests carry more weight than verbal ones.

Bring support. A family member, friend, or patient advocate can stand by you and act as a witness during conversations.

Ask for the patient advocate. Every hospital has a patient advocacy department. They are there to help you navigate the system and protect your rights. Change providers if needed. You're not obligated to keep a doctor who refuses to respect your preferences. You can switch. Document everything. Keep notes of conversations, decisions, who said what and when.

Special Considerations

For LGBTQ+ patients: Your chosen family has the same rights as your biological family. Your partner can visit even if you're not married. Medical facilities cannot discriminate.

For patients of color: You have the right to pain management. Don't let conscious or unconscious bias prevent you from receiving adequate treatment. You have the right to be heard and believed.

For non-English speakers: You have the right to a professional interpreter provided by the facility at no cost to you.

For patients with disabilities: Reasonable accommodations must be made.

The Bottom Line

You have more power than you realize:

You can make your own decisions. You have the right to refuse anything. You can choose hospice or leave the hospital. You control who visits you and who gets your information. You can also fire providers who don't respect you.

If the medical team isn't honoring your wishes, escalate: be more direct, put it in writing, bring support, request a patient advocate, file formal complaints, or change providers.

Your body. Your death. Your choice.

Know your rights. Use them.

"Knowledge is power. Knowing your rights gives you control over your own death".

PART FOUR:

MAKING IT NORMAL

CHAPTER 13:

The Last Gift Annual Review: Making Death Planning as Routine as Tax Season

---◆•●•◆---

The Family That Changed Everything

The Chen family has a tradition. After every Thanksgiving dinner, Helen Chen, now seventy-one, pulls out a folder. "Time for the death talk."

Her children groan good-naturedly. Her grandchildren, now teenagers, roll their eyes. But everyone stays at the table.

Helen walks around asking each person, "Have anyone's wishes changed this year? Any new health diagnoses? Questions about what anyone wants?" They talk for thirty minutes. Sometimes they update documents, clarify scenarios, cry, or laugh. Then Helen puts the folder away and says, "Okay, who's ready for pie?"

This has been their tradition for fifteen years.

It started the year Helen's mother died after a traumatic ICU experience where no one knew what she wanted. Helen swore, "My family will never go through that. We're going to talk about death every year until it's not scary anymore." Now it's not scary. It's normal.

When Helen's husband died suddenly three years ago, there was no confusion. No fighting. No guilt. Everyone knew exactly what he wanted because they'd reviewed it every Thanksgiving for a decade. The family gathered at the hospital. The doctor asked about his wishes. Helen opened the folder, the same folder from their Annual Reviews. "He didn't want life support. He has a DNR. Here's his advance directive, signed and witnessed."

Within two hours, life support was removed. He died peacefully, surrounded by family, exactly as he'd specified in fifteen consecutive Annual Reviews.

At his funeral, Helen's daughter Margaret said, "Dad gave us the last gift twice. First, by talking about death every year, so we weren't scared. Second, by dying exactly how he wanted, with no drama, no fighting, no what-ifs."

What Helen created is what I call **The Last Gift Annual Review**. This chapter will teach you how to implement it in your own family. This is how death planning becomes as normal as birth planning.

Why One Conversation Isn't Enough

You've read the chapters and understand why this matters. Maybe you've even had the conversation. You think: Done. I can check this off my list. But not so fast. Here's what two decades of hospice nursing have taught me: within two years, families forget more than half the details from end-of-life conversations. Consider that. You have the toughest conversation of your life. You document everything. You feel relieved. Two years later, your healthcare proxy remembers maybe half of what you said. And when crisis hits, half-remembered wishes can feel like no wishes at all. But memory isn't the only issue. Wishes change over time. What you want at fifty is different from what you want at seventy. A cancer diagnosis shifts everything. Watching a parent die on a ventilator changes your view on life support. Becoming a grandparent makes you want to fight harder. Having a stroke makes you want to fight less.

Life happens. Values change. Documents become outdated. One conversation captures a moment in time. The Last Gift Annual Review captures a lifetime.

The Difference

Let me show you two families.

One-time conversation family:

2015: Has "the talk," creates documents
2016-2024: Never discusses it again
2025: Dad has a stroke

Family pulls out a ten-year-old advance directive. Nobody remembers if it still reflects his wishes. Dad can't communicate. Family argues about what he "would have wanted."

Trauma.

Last Gift Annual Review family:

2015: Has initial conversation, creates documents
2016-2024: Reviews annually, updates as needed
2025: Dad has a stroke

Family pulls out the 2024 advance directive, reviewed six months ago at Thanksgiving. Everyone remembers exactly what he wanted because they just reviewed it. Dad can't communicate, but his wishes can. No fighting. Just following his clearly stated, recently confirmed wishes.

Grief, yes. Trauma, no.

This is why The Last Gift Annual Review exists. Not because you didn't get it right the first time, but because life keeps moving, and your death planning needs to stay current.

The Last Gift Annual Review System

Think about what you do regularly each year:

You file taxes annually. You don't file once at age thirty and forget about it. You gather documents, update information, and file again.

You get yearly physical exams. You don't see the doctor once and then consider it done. Regular checkups help catch changes early.

You review and update insurance policies when you have new kids, buy a new house, or encounter new risks.

You rebalance your investment portfolios, adjust your retirement accounts, and update your estate plans.

We accept that these tasks require ongoing maintenance. They're too important to handle once and then ignore.

Death planning is the same.

But here's what we've been told about death conversations: Have the talk. Write down your wishes once. That's it. Don't think about it again. That's not a system. That's a one-time event that goes stale. The Last Gift Annual Review changes that. It transforms death planning from a dreaded, one-time conversation into a regular family habit, awkward at first, but eventually as normal as filing taxes or decorating the Christmas tree.

The Four Components

The system has four parts working together:

1. The Initial Conversation (Chapters 5-8 covered this)

Your first in-depth discussion. All key questions asked and answered. Wishes recorded in legal advance directives. Healthcare proxy appointed. Documents distributed and stored.

This is your foundation.

2. The Annual Review (this chapter)

Dedicate one hour each year on the same date to establish a routine. Review all documents together, update them as needed, and keep family death literacy current. Normalize conversations about death. This is your regular maintenance.

3. The Documentation System (ongoing infrastructure)

Family Death Planning Folder, either physical or digital, with current copies stored securely with trusted individuals. A widely recognized storage system accessible to all in case of emergency. This is your infrastructure.

4. The Ripple Effect (long-term cultural change)

Teaching children death literacy. Modeling openness to friends. Inspiring others to start their own reviews. Driving generational change. This is your legacy.

Why Annual?

I've tested this with dozens of families. Annual is the ideal interval. Reviews happen too rarely, every five years, and things change faster than that. People forget in between reviews. Documents become outdated. Too often, every six months, it feels burdensome. Nothing changes that quickly, and people start resenting it. Annual frequency works because:

- Frequent enough to observe changes
- Infrequent enough not to be overwhelming
- Establishes a steady rhythm
- Builds sustainable habits
- Your documents are always less than twelve months old.

We already think in yearly cycles—birthdays, holidays, anniversaries. The Annual Review fits into that existing rhythm.

When To Schedule Your Review

This is one of the most important decisions you'll make. Picking the right date leads to success, while choosing the wrong date results in excuses. I've seen three approaches work consistently:

OPTION 1: Holiday Gathering

Thanksgiving, Christmas, Fourth of July, whenever your family already gathers.

The Chen family does theirs every Thanksgiving, after the meal and before dessert. People are fed, relaxed, and haven't left yet. They've set clear expectations: "Every Thanksgiving at two PM, we do our Annual Review." Thirty minutes. Then pie. It works because it's predictable, bounded, and followed by something good.

Why this works: The family is already together; no special trip is necessary. You're building on existing tradition. The holiday spirit helps soften tough topics.

The challenge: A busy day with competing priorities. Some family members might oppose it: "Don't ruin Thanksgiving!"

Make it work: Do it after the meal but before dessert. Set expectations beforehand so it's not a surprise. Keep it brief, no more than sixty minutes. Transition to something joyful immediately afterward.

OPTION 2: Significant Birthday

Your birthday. Your parents' birthday. The oldest family member's birthday.

The Martinez family reviews every year on Maria's birthday. She's sixty-eight now. She says, "Every year I turn older, we make sure I've told you what I want. Then we eat cake and celebrate that I'm still here to eat it."

Why this works: You're already contemplating mortality; birthdays signify aging. It's emotionally meaningful and easy to remember.

The challenge: The birthday person might not want to think about death on their special day. If that person dies, the date becomes emotionally charged.

Make it work: Present it as a gift: "The best birthday gift you can give me is knowing your wishes. Separate the celebration from the review; use the morning for review and the evening for the party.

OPTION 3: Dedicated Date

Pick any meaningful date and turn it into your own tradition.

The Wong family observes theirs on March fifteenth, the day Helen was diagnosed with cancer ten years ago. She survived. Now that date means: "We're alive. Let's make sure our families know what we want." They call it "Life Day."

Why this works: It's not attached to anything else, offering a blank slate. You set the date and can establish your own rituals around it.

The challenge: Requires discipline, no automatic reminders. Harder to remember without links to existing tradition.

Make it work: Pick an important date. Mark it on everyone's calendar for the next five years. Create traditions that make it feel special. Name it: "Smith Family Annual Review," "Our Death Planning Day," "Circle Completion Day."

Choose one approach. Schedule it on the calendar. Commit for at least five years; that's how long it takes for tradition to become normal.

Your First Annual Review

The first one might feel awkward. That's normal.

Here's what happens:

Two weeks prior: Send a reminder. "Our first Last Gift Annual Review is Thanksgiving at 2 PM. Please bring your advance directive if you have one. If you don't, that's okay, we'll create one together."

The Day of: Gather everyone. Start on time. Someone opens: "Thank you for being here. This might feel strange, but we're doing something important for our family."

The review itself (60-90 minutes):

Go around the table. Each person shares:

- Do you have an advance directive? If so, is it up to date?
- Have your wishes changed since we last spoke (or since you made it)?
- Are there any new health diagnoses we should be aware of?
- Any questions about what anyone else wants?

Take notes, update documents as necessary, clarify confusing sections, and answer questions.

End on a positive note: "Thank you for doing this with me. I know it wasn't easy. I feel so much better knowing we've done this together. Let's schedule next year's review right now." Then transition to something joyful, dessert, a movie, or a toast.

That's it. First one completed. It won't be perfect. You might stumble. Someone might cry. That's okay. You showed up. That's what matters.

Year Two And Beyond

The second year is easier. The fifth year feels normal. By year ten, it's just what your family does.

Each year, check:

- Have anyone's wishes changed?
- Any new health issues?
- Are all the documents still up to date?
- Does anyone have any questions?

Update what needs updating. Confirm what hasn't changed. Take a photo together. Schedule next year's review before you leave.

Over time, conversations develop. Year one is simple: "Do you want CPR?" By year five, you discuss nuances: "You said you wanted aggressive treatment. Does that still apply if you have dementia?" By year ten, you're updating based on actual health changes, not hypotheticals.

The depth grows. The trust deepens. The fear diminishes.

Special Situations

When someone has died since last year.

The Annual Review serves as both a planning and a processing tool.

Begin with acknowledgment: "Last year, Mom was here. This year she's not. Before we discuss our own wishes, let's take a moment to honor Mom and reflect on what we learned."

Ask:

- What went well with Mom's death?
- What would we do differently?
- How does her death affect our own wishes?

This turns trauma into wisdom, then continue with the usual review for everyone still alive.

When someone's health has seriously declined:

Dad has stage four cancer now. The review becomes a matter of urgency rather than speculation.

Ask: "Dad, you're dealing with cancer. This review will be different because we're not talking about 'someday'; we're focusing on specific situations you might face soon. Do you want to use this time to discuss your cancer specifically?"

Let the patient take the lead. If he wants to discuss it, spend extra time. Schedule ninety to one hundred twenty minutes instead of sixty. Update his documents immediately based on this discussion.

The Annual Review evolves. That's its strength.

Making It Stick

Establish rituals around it. The Chen family always plays Louis Armstrong's "What a Wonderful World" at the start of every review. It signals: "We're about to talk about death, but we're alive now, and life is wonderful."

The Wong family toasts with wine after their review: "To life. To death. To talking about both." Then they watch a comedy together. The contrast, serious then silly, works for them.

Find what works for your family. Then repeat it every year.

Three Generations Of Change

Let me show you what consistent Annual Reviews build over time.

Generation 1: Grandmother Helen, eighty-nine

I never discussed death with my parents. We kept my mother alive in the ICU for three months because no one knew what she wanted. She would have hated it. That trauma motivated me. I started Annual Reviews with my kids twenty years ago, every Christmas Eve after church. Year one was awkward. Year three was easier. Year five felt normal. When my husband died three years ago, we knew exactly what to do. No fighting. No guilt. We followed his wishes. The Annual Review saved my family from the trauma my mother's death caused.

Generation 2: Daughter Margaret, fifty-eight

Growing up, no one talked about death. Mom changed that after Grandma's tragic death. The first few Annual Reviews felt strange. But by year five, it felt normal. By year ten, I couldn't imagine not knowing what everyone wanted. When Dad died suddenly, I was devastated, but I wasn't traumatized. We knew his wishes and respected them. Now I do Annual Reviews with my own kids, following the same Christmas Eve tradition. They'll never experience the trauma Mom went through.

Generation 3: Granddaughter Sarah, twenty-two

My friends think I'm weird because I have a living will at twenty-two. But in my family, we've always discussed death, especially every Christmas Eve since I can remember. When Grandpa died during my freshman year of college, I understood exactly what was happening. The family wasn't fighting; we knew what he wanted and followed through. My generation tends to avoid death, pretending we'll live forever. But I'm death-wise, and when I have kids, they'll grow up the same way.

From trauma (Helen's mother) → to commitment (Helen's Annual Reviews) → to tradition (Margaret's continuation) → to normalcy (Sarah's generation).

In three generations, death went from taboo to routine. Your family can do this too.

The Ripple Effect

When you implement the Last Gift Annual Review in your family, you don't just change your family; you change culture.

Your children will openly discuss death with their spouses. Have advance directives by age twenty-five. Teach death literacy to their own children. Make sure they are not traumatized when you die; grief is natural, trauma is not. Conduct annual reviews within their families.

Your friends will notice: "How do you talk about this so easily?" "Your family has their death planning together? Can you teach me?"

Your community changes, one family at a time. Death becomes less taboo. More people prepare, leading to less trauma overall.

You become part of a movement, not through preaching, but through modeling.

The Chen family started fifteen years ago. Their friends took notice, and five other families began doing their own Annual Reviews. Those families' friends also noticed. Now, more than thirty families are participating in The Last Gift Annual Review.

That's a movement. It all started when one family chose to discuss death every Thanksgiving. Your family could be next.

Your Action Plan

Ready to start?

Action 1: Pick your date today

Holiday gathering, special birthday, or important date. Choose one and mark it on everyone's calendars for the next five years.

Action 2: Commit to five years minimum

It takes about five years for a tradition to feel normal. Don't judge success too soon. Trust the process.

Action 3: Show up every year

Even if "nothing changed," you still meet. Consistency builds culture. Showing up matters more than having new content.

Action 4: Keep it simple

Use the framework I've provided. Keep it simple. Sixty to ninety minutes. Same questions each year. Update what needs updating.

Action 5: Celebrate milestones

First review? Celebrate. Fifth anniversary? Have a big celebration. These milestones are important.

Action 6: Invite others in

When friends ask "how?" share openly. Offer to help them start their own reviews. Be part of spreading the movement.

From One Conversation To Cultural Change

The Last Gift Annual Review transforms:

One conversation → Yearly practice → Family tradition → Cultural norm → Generational wisdom

This is how change occurs. Not through mandates or fear, but through families like yours choosing to do things differently.

"The Last Gift Annual Review: One family conversation each year that could prevent trauma. Every year. For the rest of your life. Until death planning becomes as normal as birth planning".

CHAPTER 14:

Living Fully After Planning: The Freedom Death-Wise Living Gives You

—◆●◆—

Two Women, Two Lives

Maria, age sixty-seven:

Maria never talked about death. The word made her uncomfortable. When friends brought up advance directives, she'd change the subject. "I have plenty of time for that," she'd say. "Let's talk about something happier." She lived cautiously. Postponed her trip to Italy, saying, "There's always next year." Avoided tough conversations with her estranged sister because "we'll work it out eventually." Never told her children certain stories from her past because "someday, when the time is right."

At sixty-eight, Maria had a massive, unexpected stroke. Her children gathered in the ICU, unsure of what she would want. No advance directive. No healthcare proxy. No conversations to guide them. They argued. They guessed. They kept her on life support for six weeks, hoping she'd wake up. She never did.

When Maria died, her daughter discovered an old journal in her nightstand. The first page read: "Things I Want to Do Before I Die." It was from fifteen years earlier. Most of the list: Italy, reconciling with her sister, telling her children her stories, remained unchecked. Maria spent fifteen years planning to live. She never actually lived.

Helen, age sixty-eight:

When Helen turned fifty, her best friend suddenly died without warning, goodbye, or an advance directive. The family's trauma haunted her for months.

So, Helen did something unusual: she confronted her own mortality, completed advance directives, had the conversation with her husband and children, and started the Last Gift Annual Review tradition in her family.

Her husband asked, "Isn't this depressing?"

Helen said, "The opposite. I'm not afraid anymore. I know what I want. I've told you what I want. Now I can stop worrying about death and actually live." And she did.

At fifty-one, Helen quit her corporate job and became a ceramics teacher, something she'd always wanted to do but was "too scared" to try. "If I'm going to die someday anyway," she reasoned, "I might as well spend my time doing something I love."

At age fifty-five, she finally went on the trip to Japan she had been putting off.

At sixty, she reconnected with her estranged brother after their annual review made her realize: life is too short for pride.

At sixty-five, she started a Death Café in her town to help others face mortality.

At sixty-eight, Helen is thriving. She recently told her daughter, "Planning for my death was the best thing I ever did for my life. Once I stopped pretending that I'd live forever, I started living as if today matters. Because it does." Helen faced death. Then she lived fully.

The Paradox

Here's what nobody tells you about death planning: It doesn't make you morbid. It makes you free.

This chapter isn't about dying. You've already learned that. It's about living differently, boldly, and fully, because you've faced the one thing everyone else is running from. The paradox is this: When you stop pretending, you'll live forever, you finally start truly living.

What Changes After Death Planning

I've seen this transformation happen hundreds of times. People complete advance directives, have the conversations, start the Annual Review. And something shifts. Not immediately. Sometimes it takes months. But eventually, they notice changes in four areas.

1. Relationships Deepen

Before death planning, you hold grudges; there's time to resolve them later. You assume people know you love them. You avoid difficult conversations. You save important words for "someday."

After death planning, life feels too short for grudges. You say "I love you" more often. You have the hard conversations now. You tell people what they mean to you today.

Tom and his father hadn't spoken in eight years. Stupid argument. Pride on both sides. When Tom completed his advance directive, the question "Who do you want as healthcare proxy?" made him realize: If I died tomorrow, I'd die with this unresolved. That's unacceptable.

He called his father that week. They talked, cried, and reconciled.

Tom told me later, "Facing my own mortality made me realize: we don't have forever. I could die. He could die. Either way, I don't want this grudge to be the last thing between us."

Death planning makes you braver in relationships. Not reckless, braver. Because when you accept that time is finite, you stop wasting it on pride and fear.

2. Priorities Shift

Before death planning, you postpone dreams, 'after I retire." You say yes to obligations that drain you. You live according to others' expectations. You stay in jobs or relationships that don't serve you.

After death planning, you do what matters now. You give yourself permission to say no. You live according to your own values. You make changes, even hard ones.

Sarah spent fifteen years working in corporate law. Good salary, but a miserable existence. She kept thinking, "Five more years, then I'll do what I love." When she completed her advance directive, one question stopped her cold: "What makes life worth living to you?"

She wrote: "Creating art. Teaching. Being outdoors." She looked at her answer, then at her life. Corporate law wasn't on the list.

Within six months, Sarah left the firm, started teaching art to kids, and took a sixty percent pay cut. She told me, "I'd rather have thirty more years doing something meaningful than forty more years wealthy and miserable." Death planning made me ask: What am I actually doing with my finite time? Death planning clarifies what matters.

3. Anxiety Decreases

This one surprises most people. They think, "If I plan for death, won't I be anxious all the time?" The opposite is true. Before planning for death, there's an underlying anxiety about it that's never addressed and always present. You panic when someone mentions mortality. You avoid hospitals, funerals, and anything related to death. You're secretly terrified that something will happen and no one will know what to do.

After death planning, the monster has a name and a plan. You're calm when death comes up in conversation. You can attend funerals without an existential crisis. You know your family won't be guessing.

Linda had generalized anxiety for years. Death was the unspoken terror beneath everything: What if I die? What if my husband dies? What if something happens and we're not ready?

She avoided her thoughts as her anxiety worsened. Finally, her therapist asked, "What if you just... planned for it?" Linda created advance directives, had the conversation, and started the Annual Review. She told me a year later, "My death anxiety dropped by eighty percent. Not because I'm not going to die; I am. But because I'm no longer terrified of it. I know what I want. My family knows. We're ready. That certainty is incredibly calming." Death planning turns the unknown into the known. Known things are less scary.

4. Regret Prevention

Before death planning: "I'll tell them someday." "I'll do that eventually." "There's time."

After death planning: You realize there might not be time. You act accordingly.

James wanted to share stories from his childhood with his adult children about his parents, his youth, and the family history. He thought, "I'll write it all down someday."

When he finished his advance directive, it struck him: I might never reach "someday." I could have a heart attack tomorrow. These stories would die with me.

He started recording them right away. Video diary. One story every week. In two years, he had documented everything he wanted his grandchildren to learn.

When James died suddenly seven years later, his children had dozens of hours of his stories. His daughter told me, "Dad's death still hurts. But we don't have to wonder what he would've wanted us to know. He told us everything. That gift is priceless."

Death planning makes you realize: If not now, when?

The Freedom Of Acceptance

Death denial says: "I might live forever, so I'll play it safe, avoid risk, postpone dreams, stay comfortable." Death acceptance says: "I definitely won't live forever, so I'll take the risk, pursue the dream, make the change, be uncomfortable."

Death acceptance is liberation.

Margaret, fifty-two, left her emotionally abusive marriage after completing her advance directive. I had been staying because I was afraid of being alone, of starting over, of the unknown. But facing death made me realize: this is my one life. Do I want to spend it afraid? Or do I want to spend it free?

David, forty-four, began writing the book he'd always wanted to write. "After our first Annual Review, I realized I'd never 'have time.' I need to make time. Because if I die with this book still inside me, I'll die with regret."

Rosa, fifty-nine, called her estranged sister after twelve years. When I began contemplating my own death, I thought: If she died tomorrow, I would hate myself for not fixing this. So, I called her. We talked. We cried. Now we're close again. Planning for death saved our relationship.

Mark, sixty-seven, overcame his lifelong fear of death. "I spent my whole life terrified, with panic attacks whenever anyone brought it up. Finally, I faced it, created documents, had conversations, and joined a Death Café. Now I'm the calmest I've ever been. Not because I won't die, but because I'm ready. And that readiness lets me enjoy life without constant background terror."

How To Live Death-Wise

Death planning isn't the goal. Living death-wise is.

Here's what that looks like in daily practice.

1. Say What Matters Today

Don't wait for the "right moment." There might never be one. Tell the people you love that you love them today. Apologize for things that need it this week. Thank those who've impacted your life this month. Have the difficult conversation you've been avoiding now. The death-wise question: "If I died tomorrow, would I regret not saying this?" If yes, say it today.

2. Take The Trip

Life is short. Visit Italy. Stop delaying joy until "retirement," "when we can afford it," or "someday." Someday might never come.

Check your bucket list. Pick one thing you can do this year. Book it. Go.

A death-aware question: "If I died without doing this, would I regret it?" If yes, figure out how to make it happen.

3. Pursue Meaning Now

Don't postpone your dreams for "later." The well-paying corporate job that drains you? The hobby you love but never find time for? The career change you're "too old' to pursue? Ask yourself: "What makes life worth living to me?' Examine how you spend your time. If they don't align, make changes. The important question is: "If my life ended today, would I be proud of how I spent my time?" If the answer is no, then change something.

4. Forgive

Life is too short for grudges. Make a list of unresolved conflicts. Ask yourself, "Is my pride worth dying with this unresolved?" Reach out by phone, email, or letter. Even if they don't respond, you've made the effort.

The death-wise question: "If this person died tomorrow, would I regret not making peace?" If yes, extend the olive branch.

5. Live Your Values Visibly

Stop hiding who you are or what you believe. Identify your core values. Reflect on your life and see where you're compromising your values to please others. Make one change to live more authentically.

The death-wise question: "At my funeral, what do I want people to say I stood for?" Then live that way now.

6. Create Now

Write the book. Paint the painting. Start the business. Learn the language. Record the stories. Don't wait.

Identify a creative project you've been putting off. Begin it this month. Dedicate thirty minutes each week.

The death-wise question: "If I die with this project undone, will I have regrets?" If yes, start today.

Sustaining Death-Wise Living Year-Round

The Annual Review keeps death planning up to date. But death-wise living happens in the other three hundred sixty-four days, too. Here's how to make it sustainable:

Talk About Death Casually

When someone dies, whether a celebrity, a neighbor, or a public figure, use it as a natural conversation starter.

1. That reminds me, do you remember what I said I want?
2. Have you considered what you'd want in that situation?
3. Make death a normal topic, not something only discussed once a year.

Share Death-Positive Content

When you read articles, watch documentaries, and listen to stories:

1. I read this article about hospice, and it reminded me of our conversation.
2. This TED Talk about death planning was interesting. Want to watch it together?
3. Normalize the act of consuming and sharing content about death.

Model Openness

Say "died," not "passed away."
Don't change the subject when death comes up.
Share your grief openly.
Talk about mortality without fear.
Children and adults learn by observing you.

Teach Children (Age-Appropriately)

Ages 5-10: "Bodies stop working. That's dying. It's sad but natural."

Ages 10-15: "Everyone dies eventually. That's why we tell people we love them and make plans."

Ages 15-18: "Let's start discussing what you would want if something happened to you."

Ages 18+: "Time to create your first advance directive and participate in the Annual Review."

Death-wise living includes teaching the next generation.

Celebrate Milestones

First completed directive: "You did it! Proud of you."

Fifth anniversary review: Cake, photos, reflection.

Tenth anniversary: Major celebration.

Eighteen-year-old creates first directive: "Welcome to adult death planning!"

Celebrations reinforce: This is positive, not morbid.

The Annual Review As Life Check-In

Here's a secret about the Last Gift Annual Review: It's not just about death planning. It's about taking stock of your life.

Each year, when you gather to review death wishes, also ask life alignment questions.

- Are we living the way we want to?
- What needs to change?
- What matters most right now?
- What will we regret not doing?
- Who do we need to reconnect with?
- What should we be doing now instead of postponing it?

The Chen family doesn't just reflect on death wishes at Thanksgiving. They also ask: "What did we postpone this year that we should've done? What do we need to do next year before it's too late?"

Last year, that question prompted Helen to visit her childhood home before it was demolished, Margaret to finally learn the piano, and James to reconcile with an old friend.

The Annual Review reminds you: Time is limited. Make the most of it.

The Bucket List Myth

Death planning isn't about making a bucket list. You don't have to skydive, climb Everest, or travel to a hundred countries. Living with death in mind means being present in everyday moments, loving fully, speaking honestly about what matters, living according to your values, and seeking purpose over superficial experiences.

After facing his mortality, Robert didn't quit his job or go on grand adventures. Instead, he made smaller, more meaningful changes, having dinner weekly with his adult children instead of monthly, stopping phone checks during conversations, telling his wife, "I love you," every morning, writing letters to his grandchildren about his life, and volunteering at a hospice. He told me, "I thought I needed to do something big to live fully. Turns out, I just needed to be present. That was the real change."

Living with death in mind isn't about spectacular adventures; it's about intentional presence.

What My Husband Taught Me

I need to share something personal with you.

When my husband was diagnosed with end-stage renal disease, we had eight years—eight years of dialysis, decline, and hoping for a transplant that never materialized.

I watched him fight for his life with everything he had. He never lost hope. But he also never shied away from the conversation.

He told me what he wanted if he couldn't breathe on his own. He told me where he wanted to be. He expressed his wishes clearly, repeatedly, and lovingly.

He fought to stay alive and prepared for death. Both simultaneously. That taught me something important: Death planning is not about giving up on life. It's actually the opposite.

Because my husband planned for death, he freed himself to live fully. He didn't spend his final years in denial or fear. Instead, he spent them loving, laughing, making memories, and saying everything he needed to say.

When he died, I was devastated. Grief hit like a tsunami.

But I wasn't traumatized. I didn't have to wonder "Did I do the right thing?" I knew. He'd told me exactly what he wanted. We'd reviewed it annually. I honored his wishes perfectly.

That certainty during my darkest moment was his final gift to me. And here's what I learned after: His death planning didn't just prepare me for his death. It prepared me for my life after.

Because he faced mortality so honestly, I learned to do the same. Because he lived fully despite dying, I realized I could too. Planning for death freed him. Then it freed me.

That's why I wrote this book. That's why I teach the Last Gift Annual Review. That's why I'm asking you to have these conversations with the people you love. Not because death is coming— it is, for all of us. But because life is happening right now, and planning for death helps you live it fully.

Completing The Circle

This is where everything comes together:

Birth planning: Someone has prepared for your arrival with baby showers, nurseries, and birth plans.

Living intentionally: Since you've accepted mortality, you live purposefully.

Death planning: Provide clarity to your loved ones.

Dying peacefully: Your wishes are respected. No chaos. No guilt.

Next generation: The children you taught carry on the cycle.

The circle is complete when death planning becomes as routine as birth planning. When you stop pretending, you'll live forever; you start to live as if today matters. When you plan for absence, you become fully present. When you face death, you finally, fully live.

The Real Transformation

The most life-affirming action you can take is to plan for death. Because that planning forces you to ask the questions that matter.

What makes life worth living?
What would I regret not doing?
Who do I need to tell I love them?
How do I want to be remembered?
Am I living in line with my values?

These aren't questions about death. They're questions about life.

And once you answer them, you can't unlearn the answers. You have to take action. The real transformation isn't in the documents. It's in how you live after completing them.

Death planning grants you freedom from fear, permission to live boldly, clarity about what truly matters, the courage to act on that clarity, peace of mind knowing your family will be okay, and time back that was wasted on worry. You don't plan for death so you can die well. You plan for death so you can live well.

Maria spent fifteen years planning to live but never truly did. Helen faced death at fifty, then spent the next eighteen years living more fully than she had in the previous fifty. The difference? Helen stopped pretending. You can too.

Have the conversation. Create the documents. Begin the Annual Review. Then go live.

Italy is waiting. Your sister is waiting. Your grandchildren need to hear your stories. The book inside you needs to be written. The person you need to forgive is just a phone call away. Death is certain. Time is limited. What you do with your remaining days is up to you. Face death. Then live fully. That's the last gift you give yourself.

"The freedom to live fully comes from accepting you won't live forever".

PART FIVE:

GRIEF & CONTINUATION

CHAPTER 15:

Grief Without Guilt:
How The Last Gift Changes Everything

The Cereal Aisle

Three weeks after her mother died, Sarah went to the grocery store. She turned down the cereal aisle and suddenly stopped, unable to breathe. There it was, her mother's favorite cereal; the one she always bought when Sarah visited. Sarah stood there, frozen, tears streaming down her face in the middle of the grocery store. How can the world keep going when my mother is gone? A kind stranger touched her shoulder. "Are you okay?" Sarah shook her head. "My mom died. And I just... I can't believe she's gone." "I know," the stranger said softly. "My dad died last year. It comes in waves. The cereal aisle got me, too."

Sarah cried there for five minutes. Then she bought the cereal, took it home, but couldn't bring herself to eat it. Instead, she put it in the cabinet, where it still sits, unopened, a year later.

This is grief, unexpected, overwhelming, universal, and survivable. But here's what makes Sarah's grief different from many others: her grief is pure. She desperately misses her mother. She cries in cereal aisles. She keeps unopened boxes as shrines. She aches every single day. But Sarah doesn't carry guilt because she knows, absolutely knows, that she honored her mother's wishes perfectly.

They had conducted The Last Gift Annual Review for eight years. Every Thanksgiving, they discussed what Mom wanted. Each year, they updated the documents. Every year, Mom said the same thing: "If I have a stroke and the prognosis is poor, I don't want to be kept alive. Comfort care only. Let me go." When the stroke occurred, Sarah didn't have to guess; she retrieved the advance directive and read her mother's own words. She followed them precisely. Her mother died peacefully on hospice three days after the stroke, surrounded by family, exactly as she had specified. Sarah's grief is overwhelming, but it's pure. She mourns her mother's loss, not her own mistakes. She grieves because love hurts, not because she questions whether she did the right thing.

That's the difference The Last Gift makes.

The Two Types Of Grief

I need you to understand something most people don't: there are two fundamentally different grief experiences. Not stages. Not phases. Just two completely different experiences. Grief alone (painful but survivable) versus grief combined with guilt and trauma (devastating). Let me show you what I mean.

Linda's father died in the ICU after two weeks on a ventilator.

The family argued constantly. Linda wanted to withdraw support; she thought he had said he didn't want this. Her brother wanted to continue; he remembered Dad saying, "Do everything." Her sister was paralyzed, and she didn't know what to think. They argued in waiting rooms. They stopped speaking to each other. They made decisions in exhausted, grief-stricken panic. When they finally withdrew support, Linda went home and couldn't stop asking herself: Did I kill him? Did I give up too soon? What did he actually want?

Five years later, Linda is still in therapy. The grief never became just grief; it stayed contaminated with guilt, regret, family conflict, and uncertainty. She lost her father. Then she lost herself to the trauma of not knowing whether she'd failed him.

Michael's father died on hospice after three days following a massive heart attack.

The decision to stop aggressive treatment was made immediately. Why? Because they had conducted The Last Gift Annual Review every year on Dad's birthday for twelve years. Dad had been clear: "If I have a major cardiac event and the prognosis is poor, I don't want to be in

146

the ICU. I want hospice. I want to die at home. I want you kids there. I want it to be peaceful."

When the heart attack happened, Michael took out the advance directive and read it to his siblings. They all nodded in agreement: "This is exactly what Dad told us." They moved him to hospice care. He died at home three days later, surrounded by his family. Michael mourns deeply. He still does. It's been three years, and he still cries on his dad's birthday.

But when I asked him, "Do you question your decision?" he replied immediately: "Never. We did exactly what he wanted. He told us. We listened. We honored him. I miss him every day. But I don't doubt we did right."

Michael's grief is pure grief, mourning the loss, not the decision.

The Difference Is Everything

Both Linda and Michael lost their fathers and are grieving. But Linda is traumatized; Michael is at peace. Linda questions everything, while Michael remains certain. Linda's family fractured, but Michael's family bonded. Linda needed years of therapy to process her trauma, whereas Michael required grief support to handle his loss. Linda can't move forward; she's stuck in "what if." Meanwhile, Michael lives fully in his father's memory. Same loss, different preparation, entirely different grief.

What The Last Gift Prevents

Let me be very clear: The Last Gift Annual Review doesn't prevent grief. You will still cry until you can't breathe. Feel your heart breaking. Miss them in random moments, like when you're in the cereal aisle, hear a song on the radio, or during holidays. Ache with their absence. Wish desperately that they were still here. Grieve deeply and painfully for months, years, or forever. Grief is love with nowhere to go. You loved them. They're gone. It hurts. The Last Gift doesn't change that. What The Last Gift prevents is the trauma that makes grief unbearable.

It prevents guilt about decisions, like asking, 'Did I do right?' It alleviates uncertainty about their wishes, such as wondering, 'What did they want?' It helps prevent family conflict during a crisis because we often can't agree on what to do. It stops regrets about the process, like fighting when we should have been supporting each other. It prevents haunting what-ifs, such as thinking, 'What if I was wrong?' It reduces years of second-guessing, wondering if we should have done more or less. It helps avoid fractured family relationships, like not speaking to each other anymore because of what happened. It prevents complicated grief that persists, leaving you stuck and unable to heal.

What The Last Gift offers you is certainty; we honored their wishes. Peace; they told us what they wanted. Family unity; we were aligned. No regrets about decisions; we followed their plan. A clear conscience; we did what was right. Clean grief; I mourn them, not my failures. Intact family relationships; we supported each other. The ability to move forward; I can grieve and heal. The pain remains the same. The trauma differs.

Grief Is Still Hard

I don't want to sugarcoat this. Even with perfect planning, grief is devastating. You'll go through emotional turmoil, with sadness hitting unexpectedly, anger over death, loss, or perceived unfairness, guilt about unspoken or said words, numbness when you anticipate feeling everything, anxiety about your own death, and loneliness even in company.

You'll experience physical symptoms like exhaustion, insomnia, loss of appetite or overeating, chest tightness, physical pain, headaches, nausea, weakness, more frequent illnesses, and forgetting to breathe. You may also feel mentally foggy, struggle to concentrate, forget things often, have trouble making decisions, and feel like your brain isn't working. All of this is normal, even with The Last Gift. But here's the key difference: without The Last Gift, you face all these grief symptoms plus repeated thoughts of crisis decisions, waking up at three AM wondering "what if," avoiding family members, difficulty talking about the death without conflict, feeling stuck in the trauma of the crisis, and grief that can't move forward because guilt pulls you back.

With The Last Gift, you experience all the usual grief symptoms but don't dwell on your decisions because you know you did the right thing. When you wake up at three AM, you're missing them, not second-guessing yourself. Your family relationships remain strong because you supported each other. You can talk about the death without conflict because you showed them respect. You're not trapped in crisis trauma. Your grief can progress because nothing remains unresolved. Grief without guilt moves. Grief with guilt stays stuck.

The Conversation That Saved Me

When my husband died, I was devastated, completely shattered. The man I loved was gone. I cried every day for months, and I still cry sometimes. But I never once questioned whether I had honored his wishes because we had the conversation, not just once, but dozens of times over the eight years. Every time he got sick. Every time we discussed "what if."

When he died, I never once questioned if I'd done the right thing. I knew I had. He told me so. I honored his wishes fully. My grief was genuine.

Did I cry? Every day for months.

Did I miss him? Desperately. Still do.

Did I grieve? Deeper than I knew was possible.

But did I question my decisions? Never.

That certainty, during the darkest period of my life, was his final gift to me. He couldn't stop my grief, but he stopped my guilt. And that made the grief bearable.

Permission To Grieve Without Guilt

If you've finished The Last Gift Annual Review and your loved one has died, I want you to hear this: You did everything right. Despite the difficulty, the pain, the tears, and the chaos, you honored their wishes. That was all they asked for. Now you have permission to grieve as deeply as you need to. Cry in cereal aisles. Keep unopened boxes of their favorite things. Miss them forever. Feel the loss without feeling guilt. Your grief is love. It's not failure. They gave you The Last Gift. You gave them theirs. The circle is complete. Now grieve freely. Mourn the person, not your decisions.

When To Get Help

Even grief without guilt can be overwhelming. Seek professional support if you're experiencing suicidal thoughts, difficulty functioning at work or caring for yourself or your children, substance use to numb the pain, complete isolation from human connection, or persistent, intense grief that hasn't improved after twelve to eighteen months.

Where to get help: Hospice bereavement services are free for thirteen months after death, even if the person was not in hospice care. Grief counselors can be found through Psychology Today or local hospices. Support groups exist for your specific type of loss. Crisis resources are available; call or text 988 for the Suicide and Crisis Lifeline. Seeking help is not a weakness. It's wisdom.

Grief Changes, But Love Remains

Here's what I've learned from watching thousands of families grieve: Year one is intense. Raw. Overwhelming. Survival mode.

Year two remains tough. Waves of grief. Gradually adjusting. By year three and beyond, grief becomes part of you, not all of you. You can think about them without falling apart. You laugh again. You live again. But you never stop missing them. That's love. Not failure.

The key difference The Last Gift makes is that, without it, grief stays tangled with guilt. Years later, you're still asking "what if?" With it, grief can run its natural course. You integrate the loss. You carry them forward. You honor their memory by living fully, exactly what they wanted.

Rebuilding Life After Loss

Eventually, after months or years, you'll face the question: Who am I now?

Loss changes who you are. You lose your spouse, so you're no longer a wife or husband. You lose a parent, and you're an orphan even at fifty. You lose a child, and you're forever a parent, but to a child who's gone.

Rebuilding your identity is part of healing. Here's how The Last Gift helps: Because you honored their wishes, you can honor their memory by living the way they wanted—fully, without getting stuck in grief. You do this by teaching others about death planning and spreading The Last Gift, continuing their values, carrying them forward, and finding meaning in the loss. They gave you The Last Gift. Now you can pass it on to others. That's how you honor them; not by drowning in guilt, but by living the life they wanted for you.

"Grief is love with nowhere to go. The Last Gift doesn't eliminate grief; it removes guilt. You'll miss them forever, but you'll have no doubt if you honored them. That's the difference between grief, which you can survive, and trauma that gets stuck. Grieve cleanly. Mourn the person, not your choices".

CHAPTER 16:

Completing the Circle:
The Last Gift You Give

————— ◆●◆ —————

What My Husband Taught Me

I had watched hundreds of people die before my husband. I thought I understood death. But his death taught me something I couldn't learn from anyone else: death planning isn't just clinical; it's an act of love.

It's not morbid; it's the most generous thing you can do for the people you'll leave behind. It's not giving up on life; it's honoring life by accepting that it ends. When done properly, with conversations taking place, documents in order, and wishes made clear, it transforms death from a trauma into a sacred transition.

My husband battled end-stage renal disease for eight years with all his strength. He never lost hope for a transplant. He did dialysis faithfully. He took every medication. He tried every treatment. But he also prepared for death with equal dedication. He created advance directives. He updated them regularly. He had the conversations. He told me his wishes clearly, repeatedly, with love.

He did both. He fought for life and prepared for death at the same time, without contradiction. Because that's what love looks like: fighting for each day, while also getting ready for the last day. When he died, I was devastated, utterly shattered. Grief hit me like a tsunami, but I wasn't traumatized.

I didn't have to wonder "Did I do the right thing?" I knew. He'd told me exactly what he wanted. We'd reviewed it annually. I honored his wishes perfectly. That certainty, in the worst moment of my life, was his last gift to me.

After he died, I returned to work. To patients. To families. But I saw everything differently. I noticed families with advance directives, clear wishes, and annual reviews, and I recognized their grief. Painful but honest mourning.

I saw families without plans and witnessed their trauma: guilt, fighting, years of "what if?" And I thought: Everyone deserves what my husband gave me. Everyone deserves The Last Gift. That's why I wrote this book.

Why This Matters

For twenty years, I've seen families tear themselves apart because no one communicated.

I've watched adult children argue in ICU waiting rooms at three in the morning because nobody knows what Mom wanted. Siblings who stop talking because one withdrew support while the other wanted to keep going. Spouses making impossible decisions alone, haunted by uncertainty for years. Parents dying in ways they would have hated because their children were left guessing.

And every single time, I thought: This is preventable. Not the death. Death comes for all of us. But the trauma? The guilt? The fighting? The years of second-guessing? That's preventable. All it takes is conversation. Documentation. Annual reviews. The willingness to face mortality while you're healthy instead of in crisis. All it takes is The Last Gift.

My husband gave me certainty when I needed it most. His gift inspired this book. This book will inspire you. You will inspire your family. Your family will inspire your community.

One family at a time, we transform how the world views death. Not through mandates. Not through fear. Not through tragedy. But through families like yours choosing to do it differently.

Sarah from Chapter 15 began after experiencing her mother's traumatic death. Now, she hosts Death Cafés in her town. Over thirty families have shifted their perspectives because of her.

Helen from Chapter 13 started the 'Last Gift' Annual Review in her family. Now, five of her friends' families do it too. That's over thirty people practicing annual death reviews because one woman was brave enough to start.

You've read this book. Now you possess knowledge most people don't have. What will you do with it?

The Circle Completes

Let me show you how the circle works:

Birth: Someone prepared for your arrival. Baby showers, nurseries, birth plans—nine months of preparation. You were born into readiness.

Life: You lived, hopefully fully and intentionally. You faced mortality by reading this book. You accepted that life ends. You planned accordingly.

Death Planning: You've created your advance directive. You've had the conversations. You've started The Last Gift Annual Review. You've given your family certainty.

Next Generation: Your children observed you confronting death with honesty. They gained death literacy. They will develop their own directives. They will begin their own Annual Reviews. They will teach their children. The circle goes on.

The circle is complete when death planning becomes as normal as birth planning, with families discussing it openly, documents standard, children understanding death from a young age, and death approached with acceptance instead of denial.

You are part of completing that circle.

My husband didn't write this book. But this book exists because of him. Every person who reads it and creates an advance directive is spreading his gift.

Every family that starts The Last Gift Annual Review is a reflection of his wisdom living on.

Every child who grows up death-literate instead of death-terrified, that's the impact he keeps making.

He gave me The Last Gift. Now I'm passing it on to you, and you'll pass it to others.

That's how the circle completes.

Where You Started And Where You Are Now

Reflect on your starting point. When you first opened this book, death planning likely felt overwhelming, morbid, too difficult to consider, something for "later," and scary.

Now you understand: It's manageable, because you have the tools. It's practical, not morbid; it's loving. It's urgent; act today, not "later." It's necessary; silence causes trauma. It's empowering; knowledge reduces fear.

You've learned why death planning matters, how to have the conversations, what your options are, how to normalize it through annual reviews, and how to grieve without guilt. You have everything you need.

What Happens Next

Close this book. Pick up your phone. Do one thing today.

Call your parent and ask, "I want to know what you'd want if you got very sick."

Or text your spouse: "Can we talk about advance directives this week?"

Or email your siblings: "I think we need to discuss Mom and Dad's wishes."

Or download your state's advance directive forms. Fill them out and sign them.

Or schedule The Last Gift Annual Review. Pick a date. Send calendar invitations. Make a commitment.

Or tell a friend about this book. Share the idea. Plant the seed.

Just one thing. Today, not "someday." Because "someday" might never arrive.

What I Want You To Remember

Death planning isn't about dying. It's about living. It's about freedom from fear, the courage to face reality, and love that prepares for absence. It encourages conversations that prevent trauma and provides certainty that brings peace. It's about living fully because you've accepted mortality.

When you stop pretending, you'll live forever; you begin truly living as if today matters.

Because it does.

The Last Gift is more than just a document. It's the courage to face what scares you. It's love that thinks beyond yourself. It's wisdom that accepts limits. It's conversation that heals. It's certainty in the midst of chaos. It's peace during the hardest moments. It's grief without guilt.

GO

Have the conversation. Create the documents. Hold the review. Teach the children. Change the community. Live fully. Plan wisely. Die peacefully. Complete the circle.

And know this:

When your time comes, and it will come, your family will gather. They'll pull out your advance directive.

They'll read your wishes.

They'll know exactly what you wanted.

And they'll say: "We know. You told us. We'll honor you."

Then they'll do exactly that.

No fighting. No guessing. No trauma.

Just love. Just grief. Just peace.

That's The Last Gift.

That's completing the circle.

That's what changes everything.

To My Husband

Thank you for The Last Gift.

Thank you for teaching me that hope and preparation are both love.

Thank you for planning for death while fighting for life.

Thank you for saving me from trauma when I lost you.

This book is your legacy.

Your Last Gift continues in every family that reads it.

The circle completes with you. And continues because of you.

I love you. I miss you. I honor you.

Rest peacefully. Your gift lives on.

"We plan for birth because we celebrate life. We should plan for death for the same reason".

APPENDIX A:

The Last Gift Letter Template

WHAT THIS IS

The Last Gift Letter is a comprehensive document that captures your end-of-life wishes in your own words. It goes beyond standard advance directives by addressing the scenarios that matter most to you and your family.

This letter becomes the foundation of your Last Gift Annual Review (Chapter 13). You'll update it each year, ensuring your wishes stay current and clear.

HOW TO USE THIS TEMPLATE

Step 1: Read through the entire template first to see what's included.

Step 2: Answer the questions that matter most to you. You don't have to answer every single question; focus on what's important.

Step 3: Be specific. Instead of "I want to be comfortable," write "I want pain medication even if it makes me drowsy."

Step 4: Share this letter with:
- Your healthcare proxy
- Your immediate family
- Your primary care doctor
- Include a copy with your advance directive

Step 5: Review and update annually during your Last Gift Annual Review.

Step 6: Date each version and keep the most current version easily accessible.

TIPS FOR WRITING YOUR LETTER

Be conversational. Write like you're talking to your family.

Be specific. "I don't want aggressive treatment" is vague. "If I have advanced dementia and can't recognize my family, I want comfort care only; no hospitalization, no artificial nutrition" is clear.

Include the "why." Explaining your reasoning helps family understand and honor your wishes.

Address scenarios. Think about: stroke, dementia, terminal cancer, sudden accident, persistent vegetative state. What would you want in each?

Update regularly. Your wishes may change. Review annually.

THE LAST GIFT LETTER TEMPLATE

Part 1: Introduction
Date: _____
My name: _____
To my loved ones:
This letter contains my wishes for end-of-life medical care. I'm writing this while I'm healthy and thinking clearly because I want you to know exactly what I'd want if I can't speak for myself.

These are MY wishes. I know you might want something different for me, but please honor what I'm asking for. This is my Last Gift to you: the certainty that you're doing exactly what I want.

Part 2: My Healthcare Proxy
I have designated the following person as my healthcare proxy (the person who will make medical decisions if I cannot):
Primary Healthcare Proxy:
- Name: _____
- Relationship: _____
- Phone: _____
- Email: _____

Alternate Healthcare Proxy (if primary is unavailable):
- Name: _____
- Relationship: _____
- Phone: _____
- Email: _____

To my healthcare proxy: I trust you completely. Please follow the wishes in this letter, even if they're hard. Don't second-guess yourself. I'm giving you permission right now to make these decisions. I love you, and I trust you.

Part 3: My Core Values
What makes life worth living to me:
(Examples: Being able to recognize my family, being able to communicate, being independent, being pain-free, being mentally clear, being able to enjoy simple pleasures)

_____

_____

_____

What I fear most about dying:
(Examples: Being in pain, being a burden, losing my mind, being kept alive artificially, dying alone, not being able to say goodbye)

_____

_____

_____

What matters most to me at the end of life:
(Examples: Being comfortable, being at home, being surrounded by family, having control over decisions, dying naturally)

_____

_____

_____

Part 4: Specific Medical Scenarios
For each scenario below, indicate what you'd want. Be as specific as possible.

_____

SCENARIO 1: Terminal Illness (Cancer, ALS, etc.)

If I have a terminal illness with a prognosis of 6 months or less:
□ I want aggressive treatment to extend life as long as possible
□ I want limited treatment focused on quality of life
□ I want comfort care only (hospice)
□ Other: _____

Specifics:
- Regarding chemotherapy/radiation:

  _____
- Regarding hospitalization:

  _____
- Regarding artificial nutrition (feeding tube):

  _____

- Where I want to be: _____
- Who I want present: _____

Additional wishes for terminal illness:

_____
_____
_____

SCENARIO 2: Severe Stroke

If I have a severe stroke and doctors say recovery is unlikely or I'll have permanent severe disability:

□ I want all life-sustaining treatment

□ I want treatment for a defined period (specify: ___) to see if I improve

□ I want comfort care only if prognosis is poor

If I cannot:
- Recognize my family: □ Continue treatment □ Comfort care only
- Communicate: □ Continue treatment □ Comfort care only
- Feed myself: □ Continue treatment □ Comfort care only
- Live independently: □ Continue treatment □ Comfort care only

Additional wishes for stroke:

_____
_____
_____

SCENARIO 3: Advanced Dementia

If I have advanced dementia and can no longer recognize loved ones or care for myself:

□ I want all medical interventions □ I want basic care but no aggressive interventions □ I want comfort care only—no hospitalization for treatable conditions

Regarding:
- Antibiotics for infections: □ Yes □ No □ Depends:

_____
- Hospitalization: □ Yes □ No □ Only if:

_____
- Feeding tube: □ Yes □ No

162

- CPR: □ Yes □ No

Additional wishes for dementia:

_____

_____

_____

SCENARIO 4: Persistent Vegetative State

If I'm in a persistent vegetative state (unresponsive, no awareness) and doctors say meaningful recovery is extremely unlikely:
□ Continue life support indefinitely □ Continue for a trial period (specify: ___), then withdraw if no improvement □ Withdraw life support and provide comfort care
Additional wishes:

_____

_____

_____

SCENARIO 5: Sudden Accident/Cardiac Arrest

If I have a sudden accident or cardiac arrest:
Initially: □ I want all life-saving measures (CPR, ventilator, etc.) □ I want limited interventions □ DNR—Do Not Resuscitate
If treatment is successful but I'm left with severe disability: □ I want continued life support □ I want comfort care only if the prognosis for meaningful recovery is poor
Define "meaningful recovery" for me:

_____

_____

_____

Part 5: Specific Medical Interventions
Cardiopulmonary Resuscitation (CPR): □ Yes, attempt CPR □ No CPR (DNR) □ Attempt CPR but stop if not successful after ___ minutes □ Other: _____
Mechanical Ventilation (Breathing Machine): □ Yes, use if needed □ Use for trial period (specify: ___), then withdraw if no improvement □ No mechanical ventilation □ Other:

_____

Artificial Nutrition and Hydration (Feeding Tube): □ Yes, use if needed □ Use for trial period (specify: ___), then withdraw if no improvement □ No artificial nutrition/hydration □ Other:
_____

Dialysis: □ Yes, if needed □ Trial period, then discontinue if quality of life poor □ No dialysis □ Other:
_____

Antibiotics: □ Yes, treat all infections □ Treat infections unless I'm actively dying □ Comfort care only—no antibiotics at end of life □ Other: _____
Blood Transfusions: □ Yes, if needed □ Only in certain situations: _____ □ No blood transfusions □ Other:
_____

Surgery: □ Yes, if it could improve quality of life □ Only life-saving surgery □ No surgery at end of life □ Other:
_____

Part 6: Pain Management and Comfort
Regarding pain medication:
□ Keep me pain-free, even if it makes me drowsy or shortens my life
□ Keep me comfortable but alert as possible □ Minimal pain medication—I want to stay clear-headed □ Other:
_____

My definition of "comfortable":

_____

Other comfort preferences:
- Music: _____
- Visitors: _____
- Environment (quiet/lively, lights, temperature):
  _____
- Religious/spiritual support:
  _____

Part 7: Where I Want to Be

If I'm dying, I want to be:
□ At home □ In a hospital □ In a hospice facility □ I don't have a strong preference □ Other:

_____

Why this matters to me:

_____

_____

If home isn't possible, my second choice is:

_____

_____

Part 8: Who I Want Present
People I want with me at the end:

_____

_____

People I do NOT want present:

_____

Regarding children/grandchildren being present:

_____

Regarding visitors: □ I want lots of visitors □ I want only close family □ I want privacy □ Other:

_____

Part 9: Spiritual and Religious Wishes
My religious/spiritual beliefs:

_____

Spiritual support I want: □ Visit from clergy/chaplain □ Prayer □ Religious rituals □ Reading from religious texts □ None □ Other:

_____

Specific religious practices I want honored:

_____

_____

Part 10: Organ and Tissue Donation
I want to donate: □ Any needed organs and tissues □ Specific organs only: _____ □ No organ donation □ I haven't decided yet
If organ donation is possible, I want: □ Life support continued for donation purposes □ Standard protocol followed

Part 11: Funeral and Memorial Wishes
Body disposition: □ Burial □ Cremation □ Donation to medical science □ Other: _____ □ I don't have a preference
Memorial service: □ Religious funeral service □ Celebration of life □ Small private gathering □ No service □ Other:
_____

Specific requests:
_____
_____

What I want people to remember about me:
_____
_____
_____

Part 12: Messages to Loved Ones
To my spouse/partner:
_____
_____

To my children:
_____
_____

To my parents/siblings:
_____
_____

To my friends:
_____
_____

What I want you to know:
_____
_____
_____

Part 13: Final Instructions to My Healthcare Proxy
To the person making decisions for me:
I want you to know:
_____
_____

If you're unsure about a decision:
_____
_____

Permission I'm giving you:

I give you full permission to make decisions based on this letter, even if they're difficult. I trust you. Don't second-guess yourself. You're honoring me by following these wishes.

What I want you to remember:

_____

_____

_____

Part 14: Signature and Witnesses
I have written this letter while of sound mind and clear thinking. These are my true wishes.
My Signature: _____ **Date:** _____
Witnessed by:
Witness 1 Signature: _____ Date: _____
Printed Name: _____
Witness 2 Signature: _____ Date: _____
Printed Name: _____

Part 15: Annual Review Log
Keep a record of when you review and update this letter:

Date	Changes Made	Initials

Note: Review this letter annually during your Last Gift Annual Review (see Chapter 13). Update as needed. Always date new versions and destroy old ones to avoid confusion.

AFTER YOU COMPLETE THIS LETTER
1. Share copies with: □ Healthcare proxy □ Alternate healthcare proxy □ Spouse/partner □ Adult children □ Primary care doctor □ Attorney (if you have one)

2. Keep the original: □ With your advance directive documents □ In an accessible location (not a safe deposit box) □ Tell family where it's located

3. Take a photo: □ Keep a photo on your phone □ Your healthcare proxy should have a photo on their phone

4. Schedule your first Last Gift Annual Review: □ Pick a date (birthday, holiday, New Year's, etc.) □ Put it on the calendar □ Invite family to participate □ Review and update this letter

---

IMPORTANT REMINDERS

This letter works WITH your legal advance directive, not instead of it. Make sure you also have:

- Healthcare Power of Attorney (designating your proxy)
- Living Will (your medical wishes)
- DNR order (if you want one)

This letter adds detail and context to those legal documents. Together, they give your family complete clarity.

Update whenever:

- Your health changes
- Your wishes change
- Your relationships change
- Major life events occur
- At a minimum, review annually

The most current version is the valid one. Always date each version clearly and destroy old versions.

FINAL WORDS

Thank you for completing The Last Gift Letter.

By writing this, you've given your family the greatest gift: certainty in crisis.

They won't have to guess. They won't have to fight. They'll know exactly what you want.

This is love made practical.

This is The Last Gift.

Now schedule your annual review and keep this living document up to date.

Your family will thank you.

For more guidance on The Last Gift Annual Review, see Chapter 13.

ACKNOWLEDGMENTS

This book was created because my husband faced death honestly while still fighting for his life. His gift of clarity during my darkest moment inspired every word on these pages. To him, I owe my deepest thanks. You showed me that love means both hope and preparation. Your legacy continues in every family this book reaches.

To my patients and their families over twenty years of hospice nursing: You trusted me with your most vulnerable moments. You taught me what truly matters at the end of life. You showed me the difference between a good death and a traumatic one. This book is built on the lessons you shared with me. Thank you for allowing me to witness your courage, love, and humanity.

To my fellow hospice nurses, social workers, chaplains, and aides: We do sacred work. We sit with death when others look away. We hold space for grief when others offer platitudes. We advocate for peaceful deaths in a system designed for aggressive treatment. Your dedication inspires me every day. This book is for the families we serve and for us.

To the families who allowed me to share their stories in these pages: Your bravery to be open will help other families avoid trauma. The Chen family, the Martinez family, Sarah, Linda, Michael, Helen, and many others—your stories make death planning real and relatable. Thank you for trusting me.

To the death-positive movement and the pioneers before us: Dame Cicely Saunders, who established modern hospice care; Elisabeth Kübler-Ross, who taught us to talk openly about death; Atul Gawande, whose "Being Mortal" sparked vital conversations; Caitlin Doughty, whose work makes death less frightening. You paved the way. I am walking the path you cleared.

To organizations working to normalize conversations about death: Death Café, The Conversation Project, Coalition for Compassionate Care, and numerous hospice organizations nationwide, your work is essential.

You're transforming culture one conversation at a time.

To everyone who has ever sat in a hospital at 2 AM, troubled by the question "What would they have wanted?" this book is my response. I wrote it so no family has to go through that uncertainty again.

To you, the reader: Thank you for having the courage to open this book. Death planning isn't easy, but you're here, which shows you care enough about your family to confront what most people avoid. That bravery will make a difference for those you love.

And finally, to every family participating in The Last Gift Annual Review: You are part of a movement. You are making death planning as normal as birth planning. You are completing the circle. Thank you for being brave enough to start.

May we all give and receive The Last Gift.

With gratitude and hope,
Donnett

ABOUT THE AUTHOR

Donnett Sinclair, RN, MSN, MBA

Donnett Sinclair, RN, MSN, MBA, is a registered nurse with over twenty years of experience in home health and hospice care. With credentials including an MSN and MBA, she brings both clinical expertise and a systems-level understanding to the complex world of end-of-life care.

For over twenty years, Donnett has guided families through their most difficult moments. She has witnessed peaceful deaths and traumatic ones. She has seen families come together thanks to clear advance directives and others torn apart by uncertainty. She has observed patients die exactly as they wished, and others die in ways they would have hated, simply because no one asked.

These experiences revealed a harsh truth to her: the difference between a peaceful death and a traumatic one often depends on a single conversation.

When Donnett's husband, Horace, was diagnosed with End-Stage Renal Disease, she faced her own mortality in a new way. For eight years, she watched him fight for his life while also preparing for his death, demonstrating that hope and planning are not mutually exclusive but acts of love. When he died, the conversations they had over the years helped her avoid the guilt and uncertainty that haunt many grieving families.

That experience changed her from a hospice nurse who understood the importance of advance care planning into an advocate who lives it. She realized that if she, a hospice professional, struggled with denial and avoidance, then everyone else faced the same challenges. The Last Gift is the result of that realization.

This book combines Donnett's clinical expertise with her personal experience as both a hospice nurse and a widow. She writes with the authority of someone who has guided thousands through death and the vulnerability of someone who has faced profound loss herself. The result is a book that is both highly practical and deeply moving.

Donnett developed The Last Gift Annual Review™—a unique system that turns death planning from a one-time, dreaded talk into an ongoing family practice. By making death conversations a regular yearly habit, she believes families can gain the same certainty and peace her husband provided.

Her vision is bold yet simple: The Last Gift should ignite a movement where death planning becomes as routine as birth planning. Where families meet annually to review wishes with the same familiarity they have for holidays. Where children grow up death-literate instead of death-avoidant. Where no family ever again sits in a hospital at 2 AM asking, "What would they have wanted?"

This book is her contribution to that movement. She hopes it inspires readers not just to have conversations with their own families, but to spread the practice, one Annual Review at a time, one family at a time, until death planning is no longer a taboo but just something responsible adults do.

Donnett lives with the certainty her husband gave her: grief is inevitable, but trauma is preventable. This book is her gift to families everywhere, a roadmap for giving and receiving The Last Gift.

Connect with Donnett:

Website: DonnettSinclair.com

Email: donnett@donnettsinclair.com

Speaking inquiries: donnett@donnettsinclair.com

For Bulk Orders:

The Last Gift is available for bulk purchase for hospice organizations, healthcare facilities, caregiver support groups, faith communities, and professional development programs.

Contact: donnett@donnettsinclair.com

www.ingramcontent.com/pod-product-compliance
Lightning Source LLC
Chambersburg PA
CBHW021044130626
46552CB00005B/2011